# WE CAN DO I.T. TOO

## Using computers in activity programmes for people with dementia

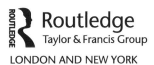

T0346296

**Nada Savitch & Verity Stokes**

Routledge
Taylor & Francis Group

LONDON AND NEW YORK

First published 2011 by Speechmark Publishing Ltd.

Published 2017 by Routledge
2 Park Square, Milton Park, Abingdon, Oxon OX14 4RN
711 Third Avenue, New York, NY 10017, USA

*Routledge is an imprint of the Taylor & Francis Group, an informa business*

**British Library cataloguing in publication data**
A catalogue record for this book is available from the British Library

ISBN 9780863888328 (pbk)

# Contents

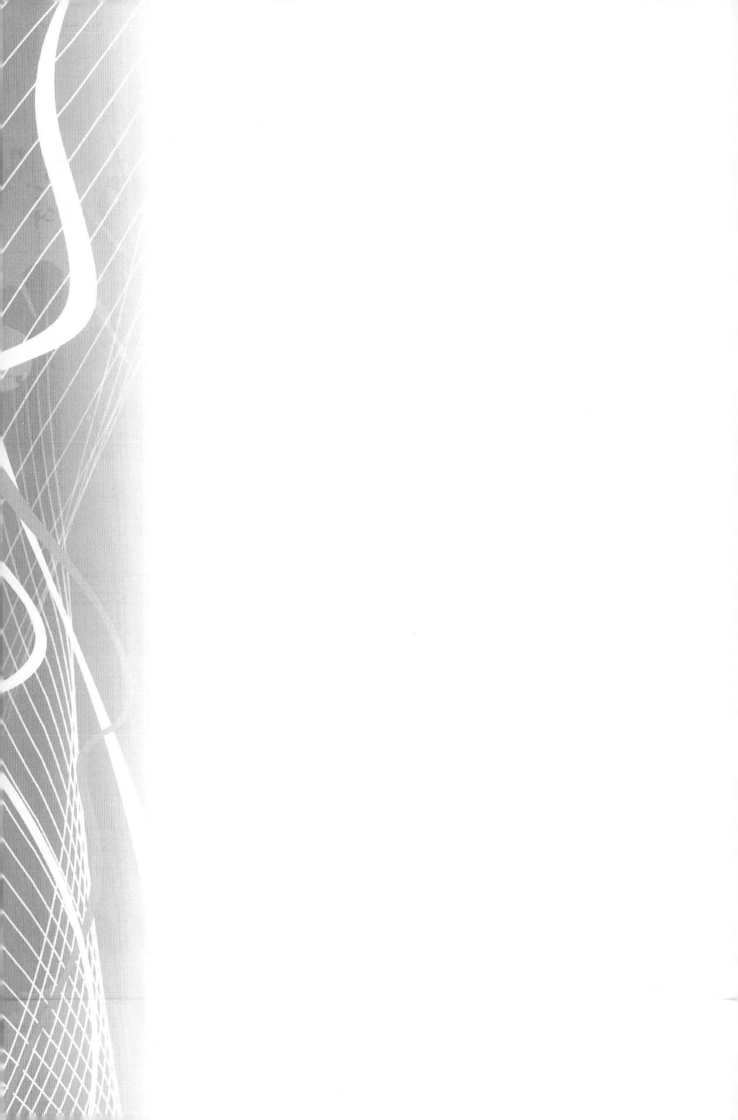

# Preface

## Verity's story

About eight years ago I was asked to be part of a small team setting up a community-based speech and language therapy service for older people with mental health difficulties in Warwickshire. I had no experience in mental health and admit I felt anxious about what to expect. I have always approached communication therapy and activities in a practical, functional way, preferring to work with people where they feel comfortable – in their own homes, at the shops or during social activities – but was unsure how I was going to work with people with significant memory difficulties. Would I have to change my practice and was I up to the job? I accepted the challenge with some trepidation, but how glad I am that I did!

I should have realised that, contrary to my preconceptions, I was working with people first and foremost, their varying diagnoses being only one small aspect of the whole person, with the same interests, hopes for the future, curiosity about new things, and rich and varied lives as we all have. I have been privileged to meet some wonderful people and their families and carers; their enthusiasm, skill and zest for life have been inspiring. Most importantly, we have laughed, made mistakes together and enjoyed learning new ways of doing things.

I started using computers and information technology (IT) in groups as an aid to instantly look up information, answer queries that arose and help people's communication. Digital photography has proved invaluable in creating a record of a trip, group or event and can be used to help people remember and describe their experiences.

## Nada's story

When I started work as website manager at the Alzheimer's Society in 2000 I had no knowledge of dementia. Rachael Litherland was running the 'Living with Dementia' programme at the Society at that time and she asked me if I would work with Peter Ashley, newly diagnosed with Lewy Body dementia. At the time I thought every team at the Society's national office was paired with someone with dementia – it was only later that I found out I was the only one! Peter is an IT expert – he has also been an inspiration to me and has now become a friend. I also became involved in a computer project run by Ellie Potier at the West Kent branch of the Alzheimer's Society. Ellie used computers with different groups of people with dementia.

When I left the Society, Rachael Litherland, Steve Milton and I founded a community interest company called Innovations in Dementia. One of our first projects was funded by NESTA (the National Endowment for Science, Technology and the Arts) and was a joint project with Housing21 Dementia Voice. The project involved working with staff at two Housing21 day centres to introduce computers and the internet as part of their activities programmes. I learned a great deal from the staff and from people with dementia at the day centres, and also from Jennie Whitford at the Alzheimer's Society in Hounslow where I volunteer at their computer club, which is open to people with dementia, carers and former carers.

## How this book came about

We first met at a branch of the Alzheimer's Society in Leamington Spa and subsequently at a conference where we realised that we shared similar experiences and interests in encouraging the use of IT with people with dementia. This book is about our shared passion for helping people with dementia to get the most out of IT. We draw on all our experience of running projects and also from the experience and ideas of the staff, volunteers and people with dementia with whom we have worked.

# How to use this book

Many people think that computers and people with dementia do not mix. As you are reading this book, you are probably not one of them! Like it or not, computers and other digital gadgets such as cameras and mobile phones are part of our lives. We believe it is important that people with dementia engage with the same activities as the rest of us.

This book is based on our real experiences and is designed to inspire people working in any dementia service. This includes care workers and managers, occupational and speech and language therapists, specialist activity workers and volunteers working in people's homes, day care centres, voluntary organisations and care homes.

We hope this book will be used to inspire people to use computers and other information technologies with people with dementia. We do not offer a step-by-step guide – instead we offer some of our experiences that we hope will give you ideas for your own work. We have provided real-life examples to illustrate most sections. These examples have come from our own experiences but the names and locations have been changed.

This book cannot be a guide to using computers as there are simply too many different versions of hardware and software. We have tried to use generic terms wherever we can and have included a glossary of terms to help you explain some of the technical words to the people you are working with. This book is not a manual or computer training course. We presume a certain level of competency in using computers, or the enthusiasm to find a course that will teach you more. Most people are self-taught when it comes to using everyday software such as for writing letters, searching the internet or creating presentations. We don't expect you – or the people with dementia you work with – to become computer experts. We just want you to have fun!

We have divided the book into three sections.

## 1 Setting up
The first section of this book provides some background information for anyone starting out. We hope that it will stop you falling into some of the traps that we did! We also hope that it will give you some ammunition when you are trying to persuade others that people with dementia and computers do mix!

### 2 Ideas

The second section aims to give you some ideas for the type of activity that can be done with the help of IT. You won't find a step-by-step guide, but we hope you will find some inspiration and some ideas that you can build on.

### 3 Practical help: examples

The third section is the most technical. We have provided a few graphic examples of some of the activities in Part 2. These are just suggestions to get you started and give you an idea of what some of the end products might look like. There is also an explanation of the types of software and techniques you might be using.

Don't read this book from cover to cover. Dip in where you want – and when you get to a brick wall and think you have no imagination left!

# Part 1 Setting up

# How to use this section

In this section we discuss some of the issues around introducing computer work to a dementia care setting. This work could be:

- a specialist group set up in the community with referrals from various sources
- an ad hoc activity in a day centre or residential home
- a new group offered to existing users of your service.

We have tried to cover the main issues to enable you to plan your service, engage the right people and get the necessary funding, and also to avoid some of the pitfalls we experienced. We have tried to give ideas about equipment without giving specific recommendations, which would not be suitable for everyone and would be out of date very quickly. We have also stressed the importance of people – management, your IT team, volunteers and the people with dementia you work with.

Like the book as a whole, this section is not intended to be read from cover to cover. Some of the issues raised may not be relevant to your situation. Glancing through the headings and reading some of the real-life stories will give you a feel for the subjects we believe are important.

# Background

According to information published online by the Alzheimer's Society, there are currently 750,000 people with dementia in the United Kingdom. In nursing homes 80 to 90% of residents have some form of dementia. There will be over a million people with dementia by 2025 (Alzheimer's Society, 2011). Someone with a physical illness is likely to need care in a residential home near the end of their life. However, people with cognitive difficulties will spend longer in this kind of setting.

Vocational training courses seldom include specific skills in engagement and communication with people who have dementia, and there is a lack of resources available. Engaging patients and their carers in dementia care services can be problematic. Whether at initial diagnosis or later on, people wonder what to expect, who they will meet and what activities will be offered to them. They often talk of a fear of sitting around in armchairs, silently staring at other people in the room, nobody speaking to anyone else or sharing ideas, opinions and jokes. They may feel self-conscious and be aware of memory and communication difficulties, or feel that there is little of interest to engage them. Sometimes their experiences will have been quite negative and there may be a reluctance to venture away from familiar surroundings where they are not under pressure to socialise and make the acquaintance of new people. A service offering something relatively new and exciting such as working with computers and other types of IT may overcome some of these obstacles.

# Who can do IT?

Everyone in your service can engage with computers at some level. The level of engagement will depend on:

- the person's interest in computers
- the relevance of what you are doing to their other interests
- their previous experience of using computers
- their level of impairment due to dementia.

You will find a vast difference in abilities and interest across the group of people you work with and you may be surprised at the skills and knowledge they have. Many will have learned to type in their working lives and people often retain this kind of 'procedural' memory. Others will associate computers with boring office work and procedures, or with being put out of work. It is important to remember that for most young people using computers is a leisure activity. It can be for older people too! Computers are very much part of our world and we should not deny people with dementia the chance to engage with them.

One type of engagement is active use of the computer such as:

- typing
- using a mouse
- using other equipment such as a camera.

People will usually need help such as a reminder to 'click' or to hold the shift key to produce a capital letter.

People can also be engaged through understanding that their choices can be carried out on the screen (and so into print), for example:

- choosing which picture to include in a slide show
- choosing the text colour and font to be used.

Another form of engagement is more passive, for example:

- singing along to music
- looking at pictures in a slide show.

Although this may not seem very different from watching television, the important difference is that someone with dementia can be in control of what they see. They can stop the singing, choose a different song or repeat one, and change the order of the pictures in a slide show.

# Why do IT?

## Encouraging people to engage with services

Many people who develop dementia will never have come across health and social care services before. Terms used in traditional services – such as day care, respite and sitting services – can be seen as stigmatising and off-putting. People with dementia may have had full and rewarding lives and will expect to continue living in that way. However, they will need support and help to do so. Many services for people with dementia have an image problem. Many have the look and feel of a primary school of 30 years ago.

Computers are part of everyday life for most people in the UK. In the very near future, people with dementia and their families will expect to see computers or MP3 players in services for people with dementia in the same way as they expect to see a television set or a CD player now. The idea of engaging with IT may be useful when trying to encourage people with dementia to attend a day centre or other service. We have found that people generally react well to the concept of attending a club or a class where they have the opportunity to try new things. Some IT activities are seen as particularly useful, for example using digital photography, email or the internet.

## Interaction with each other and carers

A computer can be a very flexible tool that can be used either as the focus of an activity or as part of other activities such as reminiscence, art, music and discussion groups.

Involvement in a group, whatever the focus, gives structure to a day or week, is a valuable opportunity to interact with others and can be an important avenue for sharing information about successful and unsuccessful strategies. Getting people together to share an occupation often reveals common interests and triggers memories and aspirations.

A computer group can also be a great leveller. We have found that in mixed groups of people with dementia, carers and former carers it is often the people with dementia who retain their typing or computer skills and help and encourage others, who may not have cognitive problems but are new to computers.

*The National Service Framework for Older People states that:*
*Older people in residential care and nursing homes and those receiving day care should be able to participate in a range of stimulating group or one to one activities. These can include reminiscence, art-therapy, news-based discussions, aromatherapy, games and quizzes, adult education and drama. Older people should be offered a choice of activities matched to their needs and preferences. An appropriate environment can also aid orientation and help to avoid visual and sensory confusion. This will involve good quality design, lighting, colour contrast and accessible accommodation.*
(Department of Health, 2001, standard 7.11)

The Happydale day centre for people with dementia has over 60 clients. It is open six days a week. On Fridays and Mondays it has special groups for people with quite severe dementia. These groups like to sing, and once a month there is a chair-based exercise class. On Wednesdays there is a group for people who have just been diagnosed. The Wednesday group often go on outings. On Saturday mornings there is a drop-in café for people with dementia and their carers.

The staff are dedicated but overstretched. Some are confident with computers and are regular YouTube and Facebook users. Others associate computers with tedious office work. Both groups find it difficult to envisage how computers will fit in with their already busy schedules. They are also unsure that the people attending the centre will have any interest in computers. In fact, many staff think the computers would be confusing and distressing for their clients.

The activities coordinator Jan was willing to give it a go. She started off slowly working one to one with Alice, who was game for anything.

One day Jan was sick and tired of hearing the same old Vera Lynn CD. She grabbed the laptop and joined the reminiscence group. She asked Alice what music was playing when she had her first kiss. Alice laughed and said, 'I don't know, but I'd like to kiss that Elvis'. Jan fired up the YouTube website and typed in 'Elvis'. Within 10 minutes the whole group was up dancing and singing.

At the end of the year Jan looked back at all the files on the computer. She found some beautiful photographs and artwork along with images of different activities and trips.

As she planned the Christmas party she thought it would be lovely to give everyone a gift. She found pictures of each group and printed them out. She bought some calendars for next year and stuck them on the bottom. Jan vowed that next year she would include clients in the development of a proper calendar for the centre.

Jan realised that people outside the day centre often didn't know what happened within. Farook had just started work at the centre. In his interview he said that he was involved in producing a newsletter for his local community group. Jan wondered if he'd be able to work with clients to produce a monthly newsletter for the centre.

Slowly the computer has become an invaluable tool for many of the activities at the day centre.

# Engagement with wider society

Computers and communications technologies are everywhere we look. Most television and radio programmes urge us to look at a website for more information, mobile phones are everywhere, taking digital photographs is commonplace. If people with dementia are excluded from this IT world they risk being cut off from much of society.

> *Zoltan has always kept in touch with his family in Poland, but since his brother died he no longer gets letters. The younger generation have no time to write, he tells Jan at the day centre. Jan investigates the possibility of using email to communicate with Zoltan's nephews.*

IT offers choice about how and when people do their hobbies. For example, watching television programmes via a computer allows people to stop watching when they get bored or distracted.

> *Fred was always interested in nature programmes on TV, but now he finds it difficult to concentrate on a 50-minute programme. Edna is upset that this small pleasure seems to be slipping away from her husband. Edna mentions this to the staff at the day centre. Monique decides to try something: she shows Fred the programme's website. Because Fred can choose what to look at, he is no longer bored. Monique prints out a long piece of text – and Fred asks if he can take it home to share with Edna.*

At day centres, much of the information – notices, menus etc. – is produced in the office. Encouraging members of the day centre to help to produce some of the documents means that they feel part of the service and have a connection with the staff.

# Gains for services

Professor Sube Banerjee wrote a Government commissioned review into the use of antipsychotic medication for people with dementia prescribed to control challenging behaviours (Banerjee, 2009). There is a Government aim to reduce the use of these drugs by one third of the current level of prescribing. However, alongside this there is an acknowledged need to improve skills and resources in primary care and to increase meaningful activities in care settings that relate to individual preferences. This would bring to both the National Health Service and individuals the benefits of decreased prescribing and increased quality of life. The Care Quality Commission's document *Equality in Later Life* found that 'meaningful activities provided that meet

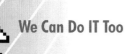

the needs of the patients' had a beneficial effect in the quality of patient care (Healthcare Commission, 2009, p5).

> *Ricky had had a stroke and was subsequently diagnosed with vascular dementia. He had communication difficulties that made it difficult for him to read or follow complex speech. He was living at home with his wife, who felt that Ricky would enjoy some independent activity. Ricky was a retired photographer who still enjoyed taking digital photographs but struggled to organise these using a computer as the written instructions were too complex for him. Ricky agreed to attend a local day centre where there was a computer that he could use. Unfortunately, there was nobody available to help Ricky with the instructions, so he was left feeling frustrated.*
>
> *A local speech and language therapy group was found that was able to support Ricky's photographic work and assist him to use the computer to load and print his photographs. Ricky made very good use of this hobby to support his communication difficulties by making visual diaries of everyday events and journeys, which he used to explain to people where he had been or what he had been doing.*

## What's in it for staff?

Many staff may think they already have enough to cope with. They are often overworked and feel that they have no time to learn new things. At the same time, many staff in day centres may feel that they too are missing out on using computers and IT. They too are bombarded with promotions about the latest gadget, camera, mobile phone or website. Using computers with their clients allows staff to increase their own knowledge and expertise. Using everyday computer software, such as the Microsoft Office programs, Word and PowerPoint, allows staff to improve their skills in a directly relevant way. Improved IT skills mean that staff are more useful to the service as a whole; they will be more confident to use IT for record keeping or other administrative tasks. Training staff to use computers may also help with staff retention: they may feel more valued, have more confidence and feel that they are learning new and important skills.

It is easy for care staff to become pigeonholed in the same routines. IT opens up a range of options: touch screen artwork, creating cards or calendars, using the web to find information or pictures, or using IT in planning. Using computers enables staff to do new things with the people they work with every day. Having a more varied working day and providing interests that are meaningful for each person can be rewarding and will enable staff to enjoy their jobs because the residents are more engaged and consequently may be less agitated (Smith *et al*, 2009).

# The importance of people

For any project or new way of working to succeed it is vitally important to think about the people involved. As you are working with people with dementia you are naturally committed to making the world a better place for them, even if just for a few hours. However, don't forget the other people you interact with.

## Getting people on your side

Since you are reading this book, you probably think that IT has a real place in services and activities for people with dementia, but you will soon realise that not everyone feels the same.

### Senior management

It is difficult to introduce any new initiative without the support of senior management. They will be interested in how cost-effective your idea is and its impact on other staff and resources. Using IT to aid activities with people with dementia is still relatively new, but the benefits are proven in terms of staff development (see the section 'Why do IT?'), the engagement of people with dementia, and marking your service as forward thinking and a good place both to attend and work in. In the environment where service user choice is to the fore, offering something different, fun and flexible marks out your service from others.

### IT staff

It is a good idea to involve your IT team from the beginning, as they may not be happy for you to use their systems. Listen to what they say and try to get answers to questions such as:

- Will they be able to help with purchasing equipment?
- Will they offer assistance with maintenance and upgrades?
- Do they know about health and safety procedures for computer equipment?
- Will you need a separate phone line for your internet connection?

### Co-workers and other staff

Co-workers may feel that introducing IT into the service is a self-indulgence on your part and possibly an excuse for you not to carry out other tasks. Try to involve as many other staff members as possible.

Most staff will have specific interests, for example in art, history or sport. This book will help you to show them examples of how they could use the IT equipment to support them in their work.

## Working with volunteers

When considering working with groups of people with memory difficulties it is important to have sufficient staff to ensure that all group members enjoy the experience, that their physical and emotional needs are met and that they are fully supported in participating in the group activities.

Volunteers can bring a wealth of experience and expertise to health and social care settings. The setting in which the group will meet will often have its own policies and procedures such as Criminal Records Bureau (CRB) check requirements. Make sure that you are familiar with these before recruiting any volunteer help. People with memory difficulties are a vulnerable group and deserve to know that their interests are protected.

Finding the right volunteer is important. There may be a group of volunteers already working in your organisation or at a local organisation such as the Alzheimer's Society that you could tap into. It is worth contacting local colleges, who may have a volunteer scheme or be running the Duke of Edinburgh award scheme. It is very useful to have someone with IT experience to call on. They will be able to give help and advice on setting up a computer, are likely to be familiar with the software and will probably enjoy problem solving all the technical issues.

> *Jane is in her thirties. She worked in IT before developing an illness that left her unable to work full-time. She spent a period of time in hospital and wanted to volunteer to help with an outpatient media group.*
>
> *Jane has been able to spend some time setting up computers in a group therapy room in the hospital. She has been attending groups for over two years and has become a valuable member. She has developed skills in talking to and encouraging individuals with their projects and is very popular with the patients. Jane has also 'befriended' patients in residential settings, after going through CRB checks and providing references, helping them to access the internet and use their personal computers.*

You will need to be clear about the role you expect your volunteer(s) to play. It may be that they are comfortable 'in the background', or they may want to take a fully active role within the group. Volunteers need to thoroughly understand and respect confidentiality rules. Invite the volunteer in to discuss how they see their role and what is expected of them well before the group meets. Perhaps they could have an opportunity to meet some of the individuals or group members informally so that they can get to know each other. It is important to remember that, while a valuable resource, volunteers cannot be expected to take on the responsibilities of employed members of staff.

> *A contact at the local branch of the Alzheimer's Society asked if Bob could volunteer to help with a group. He usually befriended people through the Society and took them out on an individual basis. Some of these individuals found it hard to understand his role, making it difficult for him to form relationships with them. Bob wanted to get to know these people through an established group so that he could find out their interests and get to know them slowly. He has been a great help and is sensitive to individual need. Both the group and Bob have benefited from his volunteer work.*

## Group management

Working with groups requires some thought. If you are starting a group in a residential or day care setting, it may be an open group with no fixed membership. Activities will be fluid and need to be chosen carefully so that there is a sense of accomplishment at the end of each session.

Sometimes it is possible to invite certain people for a specific purpose such as life story work, preparing a presentation or to focus on communication. Whatever the purpose, it is not necessary to be too concerned with the individual diagnosis of each participant as mixed groups can be extremely successful. It is usually the case that nobody in the group knows or is concerned about diagnosis and group members tend to be very supportive of each other. The most successful way of forming a group is to get to know individuals and consider whether personalities and interests will mix. For example, someone who becomes agitated and anxious would usually prefer a smaller group where they can get plenty of support in a quieter environment. Of course, there are always surprises and people find common ground in the most unexpected ways.

Some people are more comfortable with single sex groups and others enjoy mixed company. The number of people attending a group and their individual abilities need to be matched to the amount of regular support available. Make sure that there is full commitment to the group as cancellation can be disappointing and confusing.

Whatever the mix, running groups is not easy and can be a daunting task. Do not underestimate the help that may be needed or try to run a group alone unless the group members are familiar with the venue and independent with activities such as using the bathroom.

*A room at a local day centre was hired at a small cost once a week for a group of people interested in producing a leaflet about local services and places of interest that were accessible to people who needed support with their mobility and/or had memory and visual difficulties. The aim was to identify local places that could be visited with family and friends. Although there was a common aim and interest, group members included people who had been diagnosed with dementia, people who had had stroke, people who had a brain injury, and some family and carers. Each of the group members had a valuable contribution to make. Some searched the internet or talked about local knowledge, others used the word processor to produce text or scanned in photographs they had taken on family trips.*

Dementia is a progressive condition and this needs to be taken into consideration when re-forming groups for subsequent sessions and activities. It is likely that an individual's skills may have deteriorated if there is any length of time between sessions. You will need to re-evaluate each person's abilities in order to place them in a group or select the most appropriate activities.

## Confidentiality and consent

Issues of confidentiality and consent need careful consideration. If you intend to take photographs, video footage or voice recordings during individual or group sessions that show people who can be clearly identified, then consent needs to be obtained. Each individual shown or heard needs to give written consent if the materials are to be shared or published outside the group. See Part 3 for an example of a consent form.

If possible, it is a good idea to come up with a set of group 'rules' at the start of the sessions. These can be determined by the group members and will usually contain points such as respecting information shared in the group and listening to each other's opinions. However, this will not always be possible where there are people with significant memory, attention or communication difficulties. It is often the role of the group facilitator to ensure that each group member has the opportunity for appropriate input. Think about how you use photographs, the names of people in your group and their creative work. Remember that posts on the internet can potentially be seen by anyone.

If consent to share information such as photographs and video needs to be obtained, then each individual's capacity to understand the information given, and therefore be fully informed about what they are consenting to, must be assessed. The Mental Capacity Act 2005 gives sound and clear guidance about the process of gaining consent. The Act contains provisions that support people to make, or contribute to, decisions about the care or treatment they receive, even if they lack capacity. Obviously, consent from the person with dementia is vital. However, it may be appropriate and polite to keep family members and carers informed about your work and one way of doing this is to ask a family member to witness a signature on a consent form.

# IT Training

Think about your own skills and confidence in using computers. Also think about the IT skills and confidence of other staff and volunteers with whom you work. You and your colleagues have the skills to work creatively and sensitively with people with dementia. Before embarking on additional training, think about:

- what activities you are going to do
- what equipment you are going to use
- what skills there are within your organisation – your admin. staff or the cook may be keen IT enthusiasts in their spare time
- where the gaps are.

Training can be found:

- through your own organisation
- online
- at local colleges
- independently – through books or online.

The best approach is probably a combination of these.

Some factors to bear in mind when considering training are:

- price
- time commitment
- relevance – remember you will be using computers to have fun! A course that is very business orientated may not be suitable.

Whatever you decide, it is important that you practise what you have learned in order to increase your confidence. It is always worth looking for additional help online (see the following sections 'Keeping up to date with IT developments' and 'Other organisations that can help'). For example, AbilityNet has help sheets on different aspects of computer use (see 'Useful addresses and organisations' in the References section for website).

## Keeping up to date with IT developments

Information technology changes extremely quickly and as soon as one piece of equipment is purchased it is often superseded by another.

## Hardware

The most important thing to consider before replacing equipment is whether what you already have meets your needs. It is not usually necessary to update computer equipment frequently. Having a good knowledge of the operating system and finding your way around the equipment is far more important to the success of using IT with people with memory difficulties. People who have become familiar with your current computers will not necessarily adapt readily to change.

However, it is certainly worth keeping an eye on new developments in access equipment such as keyboards and mice. These tend to become cheaper as more and more people use IT. You may find that there are some very useful adaptations coming on to the market and using a search engine on the internet is a good way of keeping up to date.

## Software

You may find that your computer comes pre-loaded with most of the software you will need to run groups successfully. There is usually some form of word-processing program, a way of creating slide shows and a way of creating short movies. Photo software tends to come as part of a digital camera package and will usually be more than adequate for your needs. As a general rule, look for simple programs that have clear visual information and instructions and do not take too many steps to complete a slide show or manipulate a photograph.

## The web

There are millions of websites available that may be helpful. These range from sites offering resources for art or life story work, to commercial websites to do with heritage and family trees, and specialist dementia websites. Keeping abreast of new developments on the web does not have to be too time-consuming and may save you time and effort in the long run.

## Gadgets and mobile devices

New cameras, phones and other hand-held devices are being developed all the time. Although the trend is often to make devices smaller and more complicated with hundreds of different features, never underestimate the interest of people with dementia in new things. The iPad and iPhone developed by Apple, and other smart phones and tablets, have touch screens that seem to be more intuitive to use for many people. Many groups are developing 'apps' specifically around dementia that can be downloaded to such devices, but there are many other apps that might be appropriate for your group.

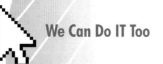 

## Other organisations that can help

However much knowledge you have about IT, the most complex aspect of introducing people to IT projects is the variance of individuals, their abilities and often complex needs. One size does not fit all! What is suitable for one person may be completely inappropriate for another.

> *Ali had a diagnosis of Parkinson's disease and Lewy Body dementia. His Parkinson's disease caused a significant tremor in his hands and he kept double hitting the keys. He had only limited experience of using a computer. Ali needed a large keyboard that was laid out in alphabetical order and used the accessibility option that ignores repeated keystrokes. An individual desktop was created using these setting for Ali.*
>
> *When Caitlin wanted to use the computer she found using a QWERTY keyboard worked better for her as she had been an administrative assistant and had retained some of her keyboard skills despite having significant memory difficulties. It was easy to swap keyboards over as they both had USB connections.*

There are local and national organisations that may be able to give help and advice to individuals who are experiencing very complex problems such as limited ability to move arms, hands or fingers in order to access a conventional keyboard.

*AbilityNet* is a national charity that helps disabled adults and children to use computers and the internet by adapting and adjusting their technology. Fact and skills sheets can be downloaded free of charge from their website (see 'Useful addresses and organisations' in the References section).

*NHS regional specialist centres advising on alternative and augmentative communication, environmental control and computer access:* regional centres funded by the NHS can assess individuals' access to computers and provide specialist equipment. They usually require referrals from health professionals such as occupational therapists or speech and language therapists.

*Allied health professionals:* local community occupational therapists or speech and language therapists may be able to provide help and advice about computer access and may have small items of equipment available on a short-term loan basis. Contact them through general practitioners (GPs) or through your local community health or social services department.

*Charities:* it is always worth looking for support from local charities, who sometimes do not have many applications to fund equipment for individuals or groups. Many charities prefer to purchase equipment that is managed by an organisation and loaned to individuals as appropriate.

Charities may be set up to benefit people with a specific diagnosis such as the Motor Neurone Disease or Stroke Associations or provide help and funding for people in need who live in a particular town or postcode area. Your local library should have a copy of the Charity Commission registration that lists all registered local and national charities (see 'Useful addresses and organisations' in the References section).

Applications can sometimes be made online or by letter. It may help to ask the group or individual to add a personal letter to support the application as this will help trustees appreciate the importance of the funding and what the benefits will be.

*Applewood day centre staff were keen to expand a computer group that they ran once a week. They already had a PC and an old printer but no internet connection. The group were keen to access the internet and felt that they needed an additional laptop so that all the members could have more regular 'hands on' experience. Sue, who organised the group, went to the library and looked up suitable local charities that they could approach. She found three in the area that might be able to help. One was specifically set up to help community projects, one to help people with health difficulties living in the local area and one to provide funding for people who had previously worked in the car industry. Sue knew that some of her group members had worked in the local car industry.*

*The group got together and made a poster with photographs, some examples of their current computer projects and some quotes from group members about why they needed new equipment. They sent the poster with applications to the three charities.*

*It took several weeks for any replies to arrive but eventually they received enough funding from the community project fund to purchase a laptop and a year's internet access using mobile broadband technology. The health charity provided money to purchase a height adjustable computer table to enable a member of the group to access the computer from his wheelchair, and the car industry charity forwarded details of another local charity who agreed to provide some computer training for Sue and the group.*

# What's in a name?

When inviting people to form a group or join an existing one it is important to consider what the group is called. If you are starting a new group with people you already work with, they should be encouraged to come up with a name. Look around at adult education courses and local adverts for inspiration.

Focusing on diagnoses with such titles as 'Dementia group' or 'MS group' may be off-putting and will not encourage people to attend. Focusing on the difficulties people are experiencing rather than a positive aim may also alienate people and give the impression that the group experience will be depressing. Names such as 'The media group' or 'Keeping in touch with family and friends' are more positive. Carers have mentioned that their relatives have been encouraged by such names and have enjoyed telling family and friends about these groups. The initial group advert or invitation can be a make or break moment for many people. It may help to encourage partners and carers to attend at first to encourage confidence.

Make the invitation clear, using plain English, and telephone people a day or two before the group is due to meet for the first time to encourage them to attend and give them an opportunity to ask any questions. (See Part 3 for an example of an invitation.)

# Finance

The costs involved in running a computer activity for people with dementia will vary depending on the existing service. Setting up a group need not be very expensive. However, a budget for equipment and consumables needs to be considered.

## Getting funding

The most important first consideration is to get approval from your management team as there will inevitably be staffing and cost implications for consumables such as printer ink and paper even if equipment costs can be sourced elsewhere. There may already be a person who is responsible for activities and a small budget available.

If you work in the public sector initial equipment funding may be obtained from hospital charity organisations. Write a clear, enthusiastic letter of request detailing the equipment required, its cost and where it can be obtained. Certain national charities may be happy to support new initiatives, or local charities can be approached in the same way as, surprisingly, some smaller charities do not get many applications for funding.

Another, often overlooked, source of funding are project initiatives supported by local organisations, ranging from the National Health Service to local councils, schools, universities and supermarkets. These will involve a process of application and will usually require some project reporting, so it is important to keep good records and receipts.

Computer equipment in offices may be frequently replaced and it is worth approaching local companies to see if they have any redundant but fully working equipment to give away. It is not always necessary to have the latest model.

If you are running a community group people may be more than happy to pay a small amount to attend and this will usually cover the cost of drinks and consumables.

## Costs

Equipment costs will involve:

- a computer or laptop
- internet set-up – make sure you have a suitable phone connection
- printer
- software – including security and antivirus.

Think about what other equipment is really necessary for what you want to do, for example a camera.

There will also be ongoing costs:

- staff training
- room hire
- refreshments.

Everyday costs will include:

- printer toner
- paper
- monthly internet connection charges
- increased electricity bills
- transport costs to and from the venue.

You may wish to subscribe to online services that involve a cost, for example:

- security services
- antivirus services
- software updates.

You may wish to use online services for specific projects, for example:

- e-cards
- family tree websites
- picture libraries.

### Staff costs

If staff are drawn away from another activity there may be a cost involved, and there may also be costs incurred in staff training.

### IT support

If your IT team cannot offer assistance, consider taking out a contract for support. Shop around – you may find a local computer shop that can help.

# Where to do IT?

Finding a room in which to hold your group or set up computer equipment can be one of the most difficult challenges. If you have no permanent space for a computer it is worth considering a laptop, which can be easily set up and stored away when not in use.

Space in hospitals, day care and residential settings is often at a premium and you may have to argue your case for the benefits of your group. Rooms in day care centres can usually be hired at a reasonable cost, or, if you are running a group in the community, it is worth investigating village and church halls as these have the added benefit of parking facilities.

Many people with dementia have sensory difficulties resulting in confused processing of information including difficulty in understanding what they are seeing or hearing. It is therefore important to consider the space where you are holding group or individual sessions very carefully. If you need to use the dining area, for instance, there will be a strong association with eating and drinking and perhaps a retained expectation of a noisy environment. Similarly, it would be difficult to compete against the chatter, hustle and bustle of a general sitting room.

If you are working with a specific group or individual, try to differentiate the area by finding a quiet corner or room. If you need to set up in a shared space, try creating a dedicated corner by using a screen. Even a couple of carefully placed flip chart stands can differentiate a quiet small area from a wider communal room.

However, in settings where you are trying to introduce computer work as a general activity there is a balance between having a separate, quiet computer room and having the computer in the main activity area. Consider the people you work with and the types of activities you intend to do. A private room will be useful for doing one-to-one work such as life story work. This is especially true if the person is reserved or likely to be distressed. A separate room might also be preferable when doing noisy activities such as singing that might disturb other people.

Bear in mind that in day care or residential settings, cutting off the computer work from the rest of the activities can mean that it is seen as something separate and different. Both staff and people with dementia might be reluctant to have a go – or think that it is not for them. Having a laptop might help as you can easily move it to the individual or group. This is sometimes preferable to asking people to move to the computer room.

Consider what you will need and how you intend the computers to be used (see also the section 'Health and safety considerations'). You will need to have room for:

- a large desk
- the computer
- a printer
- storage – for paper, printer toner, other aids etc.

### Space to get to the computer

Most computers are set up with printer and other connections that never change. You will probably need to be more flexible so make sure that you can reach the USB sockets easily. For example, you may want to attach more than one mouse, change the printer to the laptop or attach a camera. You will not want to be pulling out cables while you do this (see the next section, on equipment).

# Equipment you might need

Choosing equipment is important and a little thought in advance will help you to spend money wisely.

## The basics

### Computer

Obviously, you will need a computer and while most computers are similar, they are not all the same. Some questions to ask are:

- What software comes with the computer? There may be extra charges for word-processing and presentation software such as Microsoft Office or for security and antivirus software.
- Will it play DVDs?
- What is the sound quality like?
- What is the screen size?

*Desktop or laptop?* A desktop computer is the normal type that you see in most offices. A laptop is more flexible as it can be moved around and even used on someone's lap (consider using a lap cushion). The monitor on a desktop computer will be separate and therefore it is easier to buy a bigger screen.

### Internet connection

There are three main ways to connect to the internet: directly through a phone line, through a wireless router or through mobile broadband. Make sure the internet connection you choose will work well in your setting.

*Jan had done her homework. Although the centre had computers with internet access in the offices, her IT manager had warned her that he would not be happy for clients of the service to use his systems. Jan knew that she wanted a laptop that she could take between the different rooms of the centre. Her IT manager suggested that she get a wifi system. Because he was worried about theft and damage, the IT manager suggested putting the wifi router (the box that connects to the internet) in the office. Jan had seen the advertisement and assumed that the internet connection would be the same throughout the building. Unfortunately, it was an old building with many thick walls. The office was at one end and the room where singing activities took place was at the other. The signal between the two was often weak – meaning that they had problems with YouTube videos freezing.*

There are some useful mobile broadband packages available. A piece of equipment called a dongle can be plugged into a USB port on a laptop or desktop computer and the user pays for internet access through a monthly contract. The dongle houses a SIM card that is used to dial the internet. Check that the provider chosen has a good signal in the area where you are using the computer. The advantage of this method is that access to the internet is portable and it can be a very quick option that needs no installation.

### Printer

The printer is an essential piece of equipment. No matter what people are using the computer for, they will always want to print out something for display or to take home. Think about:

- initial cost
- speed of printing
- cost of printer toner
- whether you need it to be a scanner as well
- built-in photocopier
- quality of colour.

### Speakers

Most modern computers come with inbuilt speakers. However, if you are going to be using the computer for music or watching DVDs it may be necessary to purchase plug-in speakers.

### Back-up equipment

You will want to keep much of the work that is created by your service users. External hard drives can be purchased relatively cheaply.

You might also want to consider memory sticks, which can be easily transported, but easily lost!

You should also remember to copy files to the external drive regularly.

### Other essential equipment

Some of the essentials include:

- good adjustable lighting. Remember that if you are using a flat screen monitor or laptop it is very difficult to see what is on the screen if you are looking at it from an angle or if you are in the glare of the sun. If you want several people to focus on a monitor it is sometimes useful to dim the light so that the screen is brighter and can become the focus of attention

- a clear, uncluttered table area with a plain surface (no fancy patterned tablecloths that might be distracting)
- tables at the right height for comfortable use of a keyboard
- comfortable chairs. Some people may need chairs with arms if they find it difficult to balance when seated. However, using comfy armchairs may just encourage people to lean back and go to sleep!
- a labelled box with a lid in which to keep paper, pens, scissors and project material.

# Additional equipment

Depending on the type of work you are going to do, the following may be basic equipment for you.

### USB board

Additional equipment usually comes with USB plugs. Your computer may have many sockets but they may be positioned on the back of the machine. You can purchase a USB board that allows you to have many more USB sockets and position the board in a place that is readily accessible so that equipment can be attached and removed easily.

### Digital camera

Think about how the camera will be used: by you and the staff or by people with dementia. The fewer buttons and gadgets the better. There are cameras made for children that are tougher and can withstand being dropped or have bigger buttons. Consider taking one of your prospective users along with you to try some makes.

Think about how the camera connects to your computer; some need special software and different cables. Some computers can read the card in the camera.

### Webcam

A webcam is a tiny camera that usually sits on the top of a screen. It is most often used with voice software such as Skype that allows you to talk to someone else through the computer. The webcams allow you to see the person you are talking to and them to see you.

### Projector and screen

If you do a lot of group work, and especially if you do reminiscence or singing activities, you might consider investing in a projector that will project images on to a wall or special screen. Before purchasing one, check on the quality of the image and how quickly the projector can be set up. There may be a place where it could be permanently positioned: for example, your IT team may be able to fix it to the ceiling.

### Scanner

A scanner allows you to take a picture, photo or other document and copy it as an electronic picture file that can then be inserted into word-processed documents or presentations. Scanners are often incorporated into printers.

A scanner may be particularly useful when working with precious or old photographs. Once they have been scanned the images can be used in a number of ways.

### Laminator

A laminator is a useful piece of equipment, especially for IT projects that involve making information signs or posters. It is possible to get matt laminating sheets; glossy sheets tend to create a shine that can be difficult to read through.

## Special equipment

Some people will benefit from adapted access to a computer. They may find using a standard mouse awkward or the keyboard difficult to access because of the visibility, complexity or size of the keys. Visual difficulties can occur as a normal part of ageing or be a result of dementia. These complex difficulties can be hard to compensate for. Some people who are significantly affected will get more information from sound or touch and may have trouble understanding visual information.

### Keyboard

There are many styles and types of keyboard. They need not be expensive and it is a good idea to purchase one or two different types to try with individuals. Don't forget to check the connections for your particular computer (PS2 or USB) before purchasing anything. The kind that we have found useful are small, compact keyboards with fewer keys and alphabetic layouts for people who have little or no computer experience and are therefore not familiar with a QWERTY keyboard. Large-key keyboards that have highlighted sections – for example, vowels highlighted in a contrasting colour – and small wireless keyboards that can be positioned at varying angles are also worth considering.

Keyboard stickers or overlays can help people with reduced visual acuity. Research has shown that people find the high contrast of black on a yellow background easiest to see. There are also stickers that allow you to change the usual upper case letters on the keys to lower case. Many people find it confusing when they select an upper case letter but a lower case letter appears on screen. Also, people with visual difficulties find upper case more difficult because some graphemes look similar, for example E/F, P/R. Using coloured stickers for specific keys can be helpful. Highlighting the space bar or the 'enter' key using a contrasting colour can help people find these frequently used keys.

### Alternative mice

Using a standard mouse or touchpad can cause frustration for some people. Alternatives that we have found helpful are a large 'rollerball' or a 'trackball' mouse where the body of the mouse stays still and the curser is moved by rolling the ball situated on top of the mouse, and joysticks where the controller is gripped. For examples of these and other mouse options, visit your local computer shop or search online.

Using a coloured sticker to highlight the more frequently used left mouse key can reduce the miss hits that cause us all so much irritation!

It is possible to change the pointer size and shape through the computer's Control Panel mouse options and it is possible to set the computer to locate the pointer on the screen for you. Experiment with the options until you find what works best (for more information see the section 'Accessibility settings on your computer').

### Monitor

Try to use a large, clear monitor. This is particularly important when using computers in a group setting where several people want to look at a screen together. Many televisions can be used as computer monitors; cables to enable information to be viewed on a television screen can be purchased quite cheaply from electrical stores. If you have access to a projector, this can be invaluable in a group setting as information can then be displayed on a plain wall, making it possible to point easily to the relevant parts.

### Touch screen

A touch screen can be useful for people who are new to computers and have trouble using a mouse of any sort. There are touch screens available that you can attach to a standard computer screen. However, these are only really useful with drawing packages. Trying to carry out standard computer functions such as using menus is difficult with an add-on touch screen. Computers with touch screen monitors are becoming available and the iPad is probably the best known, but there are many others. They may become a useful tool, allowing people who have difficulty with a keyboard and mouse direct access through pointing.

## Accessibility settings on your computer

All computers will have options for changing the settings. If you are using the Windows operating system, look in the Control Panel for 'accessibility options'. Apple Macs have these options under 'universal access' found in 'system preferences'. Not all these settings will be suitable for everyone, but it is a good idea to understand what is available, for example:

- If someone often presses a key for too long and produces a string of characters, there is an option where you can get the computer to ignore repeated keystrokes.
- If someone has visual difficulties, you can change the standard display colours and sizes.
- If someone has a problem following the mouse, you can change the speed of movement.

AbilityNet has a variety of factsheets that can help with accessibility settings.

Time spent setting up your computer 'desktop' will be invaluable. Most people have far too many icons displayed on the screen, many of which are rarely used. Decide which programs you will be using and delete all the icons you do not need. These can be easily changed or replaced at a later time.

Consider the background picture or colour. It is lovely to see a favourite photo or scene when you switch on the computer, but complex backgrounds can make the icons difficult to see.

# Health and safety considerations

Health and safety considerations are becoming ever more prevalent and seemingly increasingly restrictive, but do not be put off and discouraged from trying something new. We all take acceptable and calculated risks every day and over-zealous considerations of health and safety are very restrictive.

This section is not intended to provide exhaustive guidance about health and safety issues. Your own organisation and/or the building you are using will have regulations and advice that you must follow.

## Electricity

As computers are powered by electricity, be vigilant about exposed wires, leaving computers to overheat, spilling liquids and so on. Electrical equipment usually needs to be 'portable appliance tested' (PAT) before being used. Residential homes, hospitals and day centres will have their own regulations that need to be checked.

## Chairs and desks

Health and safety guidelines for computer use exist for people working in offices. Office chairs on wheels may not be suitable for your client group. If you are working in groups, be aware of who can see the screen and whether people are stretching or sitting at an odd angle. Don't use the computers for too long – encourage people to move around.

## Trip hazards and accidents

Trailing cables can be a trip hazard so be careful when setting up and moving equipment. It is especially important to be careful when moving a laptop around. Most modern laptops have a long battery life, which means you will not have trailing cables to worry about.

Consider the environment and attempt to make it accident proof as far as possible. Think about the possibility of slips, trips and falls, sharp objects and chemicals. Fill in a risk assessment form (see Part 3 for an example; also see Health and Safety Executive, 2006) for the proposed activity environment and/or specific people attending groups. Use an accident form to record any unfortunate incidents. It is failure to record potential risks or accidents that causes the most trouble rather than the undertaking of an activity itself. Most importantly, don't be afraid to cancel a group if there are insufficient people to support it or you will leave yourself in a difficult and vulnerable position if an unfortunate event occurs.

# Getting started

Our advice is to start slowly and with something you feel confident with. It is important that people's first encounter with computers at your service is a positive one. The question you will be answering is 'What's the point?', and it may come from people with dementia, management or other staff. Computer work is not always easy and it will stretch you, other staff and people with dementia, but we think this is a good thing!

Try something that has a quick result, for example:

- drawing a picture using a simple drawing package, perhaps with a touch screen
- playing a simple game such as solitaire
- finding music through the world wide web
- making a quick slide show of pictures from last week's activity.

## Time and planning

Things always work better if you are prepared. You will not need to spend hours in preparation, but make sure that you are confident in what you plan to do. For example:

- Set up any specialist equipment before you start working with a group.
- Do a few searches on YouTube for some old favourites – see what combinations of search terms get the best results (for example, key in 'with lyrics').
- Edit the photos on the camera before you start, deleting any that you do not want to use.
- Set up any accessibility options that might be useful.

Be realistic about how long things will take. Remember that you may need to set up equipment (for example the projector) and put it away afterwards.

## Be flexible – and keep smiling!

Be flexible if activities do not turn out how you want them to. Try to learn from things that go wrong – and remember to laugh about them. Even if the computers are driving you crazy, laugh, smile and explain the problem to the people with dementia you are working with.

The next section provides some detailed ideas and examples of the types of activities you could try.

# Part 2 Ideas

**How to use this section**

**Recording people's lives**

Life story work

Recording group activities

Recording information about people and their lives now

**Making things**

Drawing pictures

Presentations

Calendars

Greetings cards

Other things to take home

Making things to improve the service environment

Signs

Menus

Newsletters

**Helping with conversations**

Aided topic discussions for people with communication difficulties

Reminiscence

Family trees

Communicating with friends and family

Email

Voice over internet (eg Skype)

Social networking and discussion forums

**Helping with planning**

Personal planning

Planning services – supporting meetings

# How to use this section

This section is full of ideas for you to build on. What you do at your service and with your group of people is up to you and you may find that some of our ideas are not appropriate for you. You may also find that you can improve on many of them. We have grouped our ideas into four broad categories: recording people's lives, making things, helping with conversations and helping with planning. Many of the ideas overlap and similar techniques and ideas will be seen throughout.

Our guiding principle is that anyone can take part in any activity. The level of participation may vary and the level of support that you need to give will also vary, but no one should be excluded from an activity simply because of the apparent severity of their dementia.

We have not given a step-by-step guide to any of these ideas; we simply give you some starting points and some things to think about. Each idea includes the same information:

- an introduction and some background to the idea
- an indication of who the activity might be suitable for, what assistance might be needed and whether it is suited to group work or one-to-one work
- the advantages of using IT for the activity; many activities can be carried out without IT, but we believe that the use of IT will help and encourage people to take part in them
- an indication of the time commitment needed
- the equipment you will need and other practical considerations
- some examples of what could go wrong
- some technical tips that may help.

We have tried to illustrate the ideas with real-life stories. These stories come directly from our experience, but exact details and names have been changed.

# Recording people's lives

There are many benefits that are increasingly recognised from recording people's past, present and future lives. Finding out past interests and details of family and friends as well as likes and dislikes promotes person-centred care. Sharing knowledge about adventures, regrets, successes, hopes and aspirations reveals the complex nature of each person's personality and encourages people to take an interest in one another. It is all too easy to respond to the effects of dementia – memory loss, restlessness and agitation – and not remember that we are all individuals with rich and full lives who can continue to be appreciated despite declining skills.

Using IT to record people's current routines and activities visually or in auditory or written form can help give a sense of time and structure, and the information can be referred to throughout the day to assist in orientating people in time and place.

People do not stop having aspirations for the future at the point of diagnosis, however bleak the prognosis may seem, so it is important to talk about future events as well as the past. These future events and ambitions may well range from simply what a good weekend consists of to a future exotic holiday or an ambition to fly an aeroplane. The likelihood or not that these events will take place should not prevent them being included in projects that record people's lives.

*Don had spent most of his working life as a taxi driver. He enjoyed many walking and coach holidays around the world with his wife. When anyone visited Don at his home, he proudly showed them his many oil paintings, a hobby he was no longer able to enjoy.*

*Don attended a day centre twice a week but was unable to talk about his interests and travels. A life story book was made with Don and his wife, using scanned photographs and digital pictures of his most precious paintings. Don selected the photographs of places he liked and remembered best, and helped arrange them with added text. He decided to include some maps of the local area so that he could point out places he had regularly driven to even if he had forgotten their names. Don found this an emotional experience and would both laugh and cry at the photographs and memories he included in his book.*

*When Don passed away two years later his family used his book at a memorial service, and relatives and friends added comments to the book about their memories of Don.*

Routledge
Taylor & Francis Group

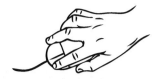

# Life story work

Life story work is a well-established technique for engaging people and their carers in conversations about past, present and future events. Life story work is not new to dementia care and the benefits are increasingly being recognised. These benefits include supporting the delivery of person-centred care and promoting better understanding of the person, leading to improved relationships between staff, patients and family carers. They also include improving the ability of staff to provide person-centred care at the end-of-life stage for people with dementia and their families, due to a better understanding of their needs.

Life story work is widely used in a number of ways in health and social care. It is a valuable way of working with people who have dementia and helps others to appreciate that individuals have a variety of interests and experiences that can be quite unexpected at times. Life story books can be a useful way of including family members, who are often grateful that their relative is being appreciated as a person and not merely seen as just another resident. Having a record of experiences, likes and dislikes is very useful when someone moves between care environments such as hospital, respite, day and residential care (Mckeown *et al*, 2006).

Life story books can help explain people's behaviour, are good reminders that individuals have led interesting and varied lives, and can help them contribute to conversations. Life story books can also help interaction between care staff and other residents in care settings. They are a valuable communication tool for people who are finding it difficult to communicate and can highlight shared interests or give information to help service or personal planning.

## Who is it useful for?

People with a whole range of memory difficulties of varying severity can engage with this activity.

- People with more ability and interest will be able to plan their own life story books and create them with some support.

- Those who are less confident may need a more flexible approach where different aspects of their lives are discussed.

- Others may want to participate by making simple choices between images or designs.

Some people will be able to select photos and materials independently to include in their life story book. They may, with prompting, be able to create a timeline of events and put them in the correct sequence. With some help, they should be able to use the internet to search for information and illustrations and locate significant places on maps and atlases. Other people will need more assistance.

This activity is particularly suited to work with individuals, although there are pre-prepared formats on the market that can facilitate life story work in groups.

> *The care worker sat with Ahmed and talked about his life and his aspirations for the future. They chose main topics together. Ahmed enjoys typing with two fingers, but doesn't use the mouse. He can put keywords into Google and is very keen to choose appropriate colours and text fonts for different pages.*

> *Jane has limited communication and is wary of the computer. She becomes very animated when looking at pictures of dogs. Patrick found this out by looking at magazines, and then looked on the internet for more pictures. Patrick found out that Jane has a pet greyhound and asked Jane's daughter if she could find a picture of Jane and her dog to include in the life story book. Jane chose pictures and designs and the end product was emailed to her sister in Australia.*

## Why use IT?

- A computer is a flexible tool.
- Pages can be changed easily.
- Valuable photos can be scanned and returned.
- You have quick access to relevant images, giving immediate feedback.
- Choices can be made by participants.
- Results can easily be shared with friends and relatives via email.
- A document can be wholly or partially printed.
- By using presentation software the book can be set up to jump easily between topics and pages rather than being read straight through.
- A life story book can be expanded or contracted easily.
- It can incorporate media such as sound/video/scanned images.

## How long will this activity take?

To complete a life story book will take a minimum of six one-to-one sessions. However, a completed book should not be seen as the only aim of the session. To have enjoyed one session and created one page around a particular event or topic is a successful outcome.

 **R** Routledge
Taylor & Francis Group

## What will you need?

*Essential:*

PC or laptop

Software that enables you to add text and images such as Microsoft Word or PowerPoint

Any specific hardware or software that is needed by the individual you are working with (see the section 'Special equipment' in Part 1)

Someone with an interest in and/or purpose for creating a life story book

Dedicated time to support them

Time to plan the activity and time to talk with the participant before computer work starts

*Desirable:*

Scanner – useful for scanning in photographs

Digital camera – for photos of people, places and participants' artwork

Internet connection – find images using Google

Somewhere quiet

## What could go wrong?

Some people may be reluctant or confused by the computer, even if they have used one before. To start off a conversation, be prepared to use other prompts besides the computer such as magazines, maps or objects.

People may not remember what might be considered to be significant events in their lives such as weddings or holidays. Be prepared to be flexible about topics. Don't worry about whether information that is 'remembered' is accurate; engagement in the activity is far more important.

Some topics or events may be sensitive and people may experience a range of emotions, both positive and negative.

## Technical tips

When producing a long book with many topics, we have found using presentation software such PowerPoint helpful. The animation function allows you to jump from an index page to different sections. If you are using images, PowerPoint allows you to move, crop and resize them easily. If you are more comfortable using Word, create a textbox first and paste the image into it. This makes moving and resizing the image easier.

A word-processing package such as Word is more appropriate if the person you are working with is happier using text or has previous experience of this software. If they would prefer to have more images and sound in their life story book, then presentation software such as PowerPoint may be easy for them to use or understand.

 Routledge
Taylor & Francis Group

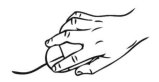

# Recording group activities

Most services provide interesting activities and events ranging from gardening or baking days, to trips out and inviting visitors to the group. Using IT can be a good way of recording these activities in order to:

- remind group members about the activities they have taken part in
- inform friends and family of what happens at the service
- persuade senior managers and/or funders of the importance of the service.

## Who is it useful for?

When the activity you are recording is a group activity it is important to involve the whole group in how it is recorded. It might be useful to talk through ideas at the beginning. As we have discussed before, how people are involved will depend on their interests and skills. It might be useful to have a camera to hand that anyone can use, or it might be appropriate to assign the role of photographer to one person for the day.

It is important that the final product is viewed and reviewed by the whole group. Even if people have not been involved in the technical production of the report or presentation, it is good to encourage them to have an input into the design, colours and so on.

*At Maple Road day centre there is a lovely garden where the group works. Everyone enjoys getting out in all weathers. Philip likes using the camera – so they decided to make a gardening diary for the group. Each month they dedicated one day to recording what was happening in the garden. Philip took pictures while Siobhan interviewed people about the work in the garden that month. The activities co-ordinator at the group supported this and helped Philip, Siobhan and Carol to create a PowerPoint presentation – with a new slide for each month. They printed the slide out on the colour printer and displayed it on the wall next to the tool cupboard.*

*The group decided that they would like to visit a local garden and garden centre. Carol found the website and used the projector so that the whole group could see. They used the website to plan their visit for the next week. They downloaded a map and planned a route and looked at the shop to decide what bedding plants to buy.*

## Why use IT?

Traditional ways of recording events or activities might include scrapbooks or diaries. Using IT means:

- The record can be made immediately or during the activity – no waiting for photos to be developed.
- The accounts can be easily shared – via email or the web – with family and friends.
- Each account can be customised for each person involved.

## How long will this activity take?

It is useful to start recording during the activity itself. A simple presentation of four or five slides of a gardening afternoon might take a couple of hours to produce. A more complex film show will take much longer.

Think also about the preparation time:

- planning how to record the activity
- assigning tasks to different group members
- researching the activity or place to be visited.

## What will you need?

It depends on how you want to make the lasting record, but think about using:

- a digital camera
- a voice recorder
- a notebook to record people's thoughts and experiences
- a video camera
- the internet to obtain background information and/or images of places or people.

You will also need:

- a computer
- a good-quality printer to allow you to print the final product to share with family, friends, other staff or funders
- time to plan and record without distracting from the main activity.

## What could go wrong?

Consent is a big issue when recording activities. It is especially important to ask permission when you are taking someone's photograph.

Routledge Taylor & Francis Group

It is also important to think about what will happen to the end product, for example your presentation. If you give it to a funding organisation they might show it more widely than you expect. You must be confident that the people involved in the presentation are happy for their names and images to be shared.

## Technical tips

There are various types of software that could be used, from word-processing packages to create a diary to movie-making software for creating a film show.

Your choice of software will be determined by the following considerations:

- The balance between text, images and film: if you are mostly dealing with text a word-processing package will be the best choice. Presentation software such as PowerPoint is good for a slide show with lots of still images. If you are feeling ambitious, you could use film and a movie-making package.

- The interests and skill levels of the people you are working with: remember that people can be engaged at different levels, from choosing designs to taking photos or typing out text.

- What you plan to do with the final product: for example, a word-processing package might be more appropriate if you want to keep an ongoing diary for the service. PowerPoint might be useful for producing individual pages that can be printed and displayed on the walls.

# Recording information about people and their lives now

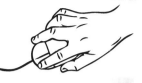

There are lots of ways of recording current information: writing diaries, video footage, photographs and timetables are a few examples. You can make some simple pages that record information about favourite foods, activities or preferences that can be extremely useful either as a potential communication chart during everyday activities such as washing, dressing and mealtimes, or when planning meals or future trips.

You can record significant events or activities. You can advertise future events by creating simple posters to be displayed in public areas. A number of people could contribute to a record of an event such as a fete.

The aims of recording current information are:

- to make a very simple record of likes and dislikes
- to prompt memory
- to aid communication between clients and carers
- to give information to carers
- to easily transfer information to other environments such as hospital or day centres
- to verify changing tastes.

## Who is it useful for?

This activity can be used with people individually or in small groups. It is very flexible and could be particularly useful for people with significant communication and/or memory difficulties; it could also be used with people who need only minimal support with word processing.

The most confident participants may be comfortable creating a diary or record of the day's events using a word processor. Participants may work in pairs to prompt each other and record different memories and may need reminding about particular events. A digital recorder could be used to capture individual stories or conversations, which could be added as a 'voice over' to photograph slide shows.

If people need more prompting, consider creating a template on the screen or copying an example (see Part 3). Participants may need some support with computer functions such as cutting and pasting pictures or inputting text, but will enjoy following your example and having a go themselves.

Other people will be able to select from a small range of options presented to them such as choosing specific photographs or deciding where to place pictures and text.

Routledge
Taylor & Francis Group

They may show a particular interest in one subject that could be included as part of a group project or form a simple printed record of an event.

> Jan knew that Rosa's family were considering care home options and that soon she wouldn't be attending the day centre. Jan and her colleagues had got to know Rosa well and were concerned that she would have problems adjusting to life in a care home.
>
> Although Rosa had never been interested in the computer activities before, Jan thought that creating an 'identity book' for Rosa would be useful for the staff at the care home. Jan concentrated on the things that Rosa enjoyed at the day care centre: she asked Rosa to help her choose pictures of her favourite cakes and drinks, she found some photos of Rosa taking part in bingo and quizzes, she worked with Rosa to put ticks and crosses next to pictures of different activities and interests. Rosa particularly enjoyed adding a big red cross to a picture of football!
>
> Jan printed out 'Rosa's book – about me' and gave a copy to Rosa's granddaughter so that she could make more copies to give to care home staff.

## Why use IT?

- Single pages are simple to construct.
- Fonts can be easily changed or enlarged to cater for individual visual ability.
- Contrasting colours can be selected.
- Pictures or symbols can be used.
- Pages can be individually designed or altered to take account of changing events or tastes.
- Work can be saved or duplicated.
- Information can easily be recorded in care plans and files.

## How long will this activity take?

Depending on the final product, this type of activity can be done in short sessions. A diary could be completed every day or every week. An 'identity book' could be added to on an ad hoc basis.

## What will you need?

*Essential:*

PC or laptop

Software that enables you to add text and images such as PowerPoint or Word

Any specific hardware or software that is needed by the individual you are working with (see the section 'Equipment you might need' in Part 1)

Enough time dedicated to support people

Some objects related to the subject being recorded such as a tea or coffee cup

Time to plan the activity and time to talk with the participant before computer work starts

*Desirable:*

Digital camera – for photos of people or objects such as a minibus, hairbrush, CDs

Magazines – good for finding pictures of television celebrities or food

Internet connection – find images using Google

Good-quality paper or card

Laminator

Somewhere quiet

## What could go wrong?

People may not recognise pictures or symbols and may become confused by pages that are too busy or coloured. Check that participants understand what the pictures are referring to and have a range for them to choose from.

People's taste may have changed significantly, so be ready to assist them in making choices even when these are unexpected. Sometimes people confuse closely related items or people such as cat/dog, daughter/wife, milk/juice.

## Technical tips

Try not to put too much information on one page and clearly separate pictures into boxes.

Use matt laminating sheets that do not have a glossy shine. Creating a simple coloured border around pages gives meaning to the message.

 Routledge
Taylor & Francis Group

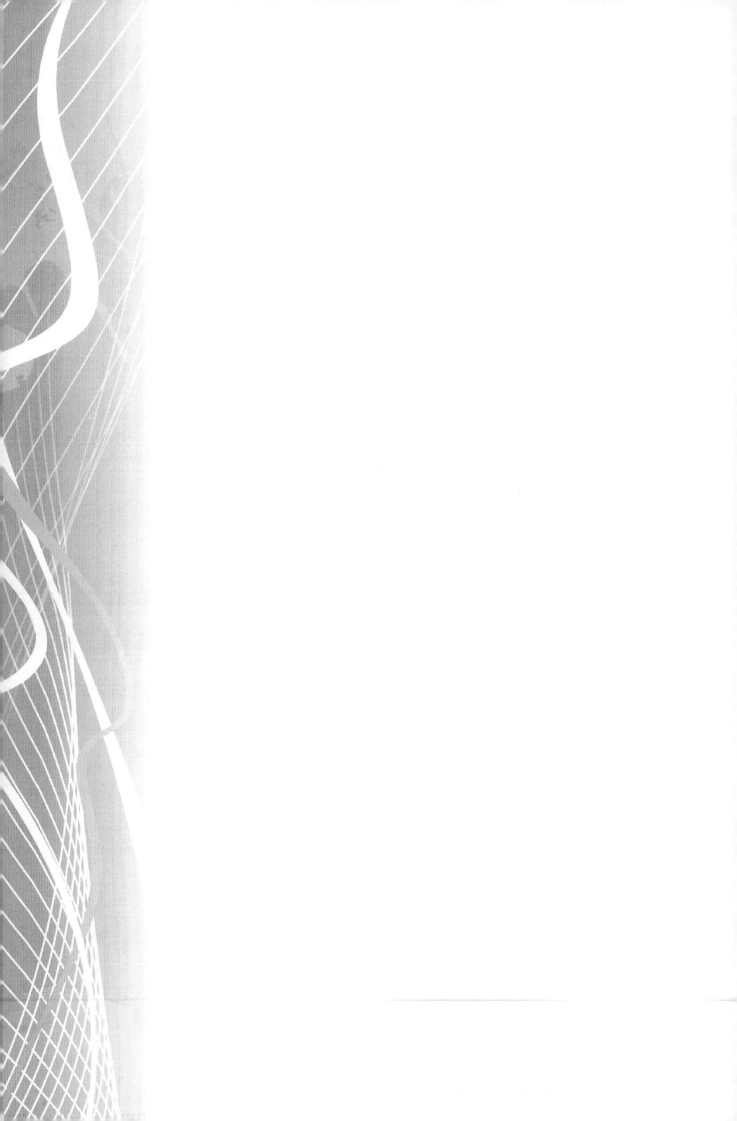

# Making things

Everyone enjoys making things. We have all experienced the sense of achievement of holding something in our hands that we have created. Computer technology can be used together with traditional arts and crafts activities.

This section will cover ideas for creating:

- presentations
- calendars, cards and other items to take home
- items to use within your group, centre or setting such as signs, menus, maps
- newsletters or news sheets to tell other people what your group is doing.

## Why use IT?

Using IT for making things has some advantages over traditional craft methods:

- Ideas that have worked can be saved and re-used with someone else.
- Multiple copies can be made easily for display and to take home.
- Family and friends who live far away can be sent electronic items via email.
- You can create a store of images that can be used again and again. For example, if someone creates a beautiful picture of a flower, it can be saved and used again in other activities.

## Technical tips

Not everyone will be able to understand what the finished product will look like, so if you are creating something on paper, it is a good idea to print parts out as you go along.

If you are creating a presentation or show for the screen, have a sample presentation to show to people.

The colour on the screen may not be exactly the same as the colour that is printed. This is especially likely with cheaper printers.

*Jan is the arts and crafts worker at a day centre for people with dementia. She works regularly with Nadia, Mary and Petra. They love the feel of collage materials such as glitter and felt. Jan was reluctant to use the computer with this group, but one day Petra seemed intrigued as the printer churned out some artwork created by someone else. Jan did not want to split up the group, who work well together and enjoy each other's company.*

*She hit on a great compromise. She showed Petra how to find/create outline shapes – for example, of butterflies – on the computer. She printed these outlines out and gave them to the group to decorate with collage materials.*

Routledge
Taylor & Francis Group

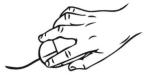

# Drawing pictures

We have found that a good way to introduce someone to a computer is to use it to draw pictures. This can help people to understand about commands and the relationship between the mouse and the screen.

## Who is it useful for?

Ideally, computer work should be introduced on a one-to-one basis but it can also be done in small groups as long as everyone can see the screen. Drawing pictures is a good way to ascertain whether someone needs a special mouse or changed accessibility settings.

> *Annie was keen to try anything but thought computers weren't 'for her'. Jan thought she'd be OK once she got started, but couldn't begin to explain the internet. Using a track ball mouse, Jan opened up 'Paint' and asked Annie to choose a colour. She then helped her to draw an outline, change the colour and fill the circle. Annie was amazed at how quickly she'd created something on the screen – but even happier when she did something she didn't like and Jan simply clicked the 'undo' button to remove it. Annie thought it was 'magic'.*

## Why use IT?

- Although drawing may be easier on paper, it is a great introduction to the computer.
- It is good practice for using a mouse.
- There are special drawing packages that allow people to create and fill perfect shapes such as circles or stars.
- Mistakes can be easily removed – in addition to 'undo' most drawing packages have an eraser function.
- Artwork can be saved and finished later.
- Colours can be easily changed.

## How long will this activity take?

Artwork can be produced very quickly and if the computer is set up and ready to go a simple picture can be drawn and printed in less than half an hour.

### What will you need?

Computer

A suitable package – Microsoft Office has a drawing package

Good-quality colour printer – cheap ones do not reproduce colours well

Any special equipment or accessibility settings appropriate for the individual you are working with (see the section 'Equipment you might need' in Part 1)

Look for specialist software that is often developed for children or people with learning disabilities

### What could go wrong?

Free drawing requires some mouse control and some people have problems with a standard mouse. Investigate all the ways to produce standard shapes easily.

People who are very good at artwork on paper may be disappointed with the results from the computer.

### Technical tips

When starting out, a dual control method might be helpful. Plug in an additional mouse for you to use. This means that you can select the colour and all the person you are working with has to do is draw the line or shape.

Routledge
Taylor & Francis Group

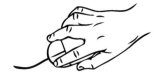

# Presentations

Individual or group presentations can be used in a variety of ways. Individuals may have specific interests but lack the confidence to talk to a group of people. Presentations using the computer can be a very good tool to increase individuals' confidence and share interests, knowledge and experience. The amount of speaking involved can be minimal. Participants can tell their story through a series of photographs, pictures, text and music, and can pre-record a commentary or speak at an event, depending on what they feel comfortable with.

Presentations can be used to enhance group members' understanding of each other. They can also be useful to demonstrate effective participation and person-centred care to commissioners and funders.

The only limits to subjects suitable for a presentation are your imagination and the interests of the people you are working with. Our groups have produced presentations on topics ranging from meteorology to local history. You can also use presentations to plan or describe new projects not necessarily related to IT. There is no limit to the subjects that can be made into a presentation format. A presentation can be a good illustration of interest in a collective cause, such as making a new garden, and can make use of a whole range of media.

The aims of producing a presentation may be to:

- work collectively on a project with a shared aim
- increase confidence
- demonstrate a proposed project
- secure funding
- encourage individual expression
- share information and encourage appreciation of each other's interests and ideas.

## Who is it useful for?

This activity is suitable for individuals or groups. As with all activities, there are many levels of inclusion, but this activity is particularly suitable for those with moderate memory difficulties. It can be used with people with a significant degree of language impairment and those for whom English is a second language.

The activity is particularly useful for encouraging group cohesion. It can be a good way to increase interaction within a group or help integrate a new member.

*James had a real interest in the weather. He had always followed local and national weather information using technical equipment that he had set up in his home. James was now finding it difficult to use this equipment and he struggled to express his life-long interest to the rest of the group.*

*James was able to select interesting pictures related to his hobby from the internet. These included pictures of the type of equipment he had set up at home as well as illustrations of varying weather conditions. James really enjoyed collating these into a presentation that he showed to the rest of the group. He needed some support with cutting and pasting, but independently decided on the order of the illustrations.*

*James found that, even though he was using illustrations alone and no text, he could still convey his interest and how diverse this subject is. He was able to use his computer skills to move through the images independently.*

People who require more prompting will still be able to enjoy being involved with selecting subjects to present, and choosing illustrations and designs.

There are many different activities that form part of a presentation. Participants who need full assistance may still be able to choose or respond to photographs and music used as part of the presentation.

*As part of a project to present photographs they had taken on trips out during the summer, group members were asked to bring in their favourite piece of music. Tulani was finding it difficult to follow the process of constructing the slide show but really enjoyed listening to the music selected by each group member. Tulani's wife said that every time he heard these pieces of music he got a lot of pleasure from listening to them, even though he could not remember where he had heard them before.*

*Maria was born in Italy. She enjoyed a happy rural childhood in an area with many local customs. Maria moved to Britain following her marriage but often looked back on her years in Italy and the many interesting and enjoyable times she had there.*

*Maria was beginning to experience memory difficulties but remembered her early years well. She attended a group at a local day centre and worked on an individual presentation based on Italian customs and games she remembered*

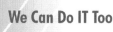

*from her childhood. She included the Italian flag, a map of the region she was born in and some pictures she found on the internet.*

*Maria needed assistance to put these on to a slide show. She managed to find an Italian nursery rhyme she had sung as a child, which was added to it. With help, Maria typed out as much of the song as she could remember and presented her show to a small group.*

*Maria sang the song to the group and managed to teach people some of the words. It was a very enjoyable event that helped Maria integrate into the group.*

## Why use IT?

Formerly, presentations used a variety of media such as flip charts and overhead projectors with sheets that required a high degree of sequencing and organisational skills to ensure they were used in the correct order. Furthermore, people needed to be confident speakers who could stand in front of an audience and clearly get their message across.

Increasingly sophisticated technology has made the whole process much easier. Using presentation software allows people to use a mix of text, pictures, video footage, photographs, animation, sound and music to deliver a report or illustrate ideas, completed projects or future plans.

People can pre-record as little or as much information as they like in order to reduce the pressure on the day to stand in front of an audience and remember what they wanted to say.

## How long will this activity take?

Presentations take a long time and benefit from thorough planning. At least six group sessions will be needed to construct a small presentation and longer will be required for rehearsal if group members are to present in front of an audience.

## What will you need?

*Essential:*

PC or laptop (a laptop is necessary if using the completed presentation off-site)

Presentation software or slide show capabilities

Someone with previous experience of the software

Projector compatible with the computer

*Desirable:*

Digital camera – it is really nice to record the construction of a presentation or any group activity. The photographs can then form part of the presentation itself or be used to promote this activity to other people.

Internet connection – may be useful to search for illustrations if you want to reduce the amount of text, but this will not always be necessary and will depend on the level of ability of your group members.

## What could go wrong?

Don't be over-ambitious when deciding the length of a presentation; keeping it short and manageable is the best policy.

People with significant memory difficulties will find it difficult to retain information from one week to the next or if there is a significant gap between group sessions.

## Technical tips

If your group or an individual you are working with wants to make a formal presentation, you will need to attach the computer to a projector. When attaching a laptop to a projector, read the instructions that come with the projector carefully. These are usually very specific and need to be followed exactly.

Laptop settings may need to be changed by using the function (F) keys so that the presentation on the screen can be viewed through the projector. There are usually three options: viewing through laptop only, viewing through projector only or viewing through laptop and projector simultaneously. To find out the specific function key to use, refer to the computer manufacturer's instructions.

Routledge
Taylor & Francis Group

## Calendars

Calendars have many uses:

- as gifts for friends and relatives
- as a way to promote or fundraise for your group or service
- to help individuals remember important dates
- as a means of communication and record keeping between your service, your client and their family or carers.

### Who is it useful for?

People with different abilities will have different input into calendar making. They can be involved in choosing designs and colour schemes, adding pictures, or adding information that is important to them.

If you are part of a wider service such as a day care centre it might be useful to make individual monthly calendars or diaries for each person. These could include days when the person attends the group, details of planned activities for the month and other important dates such as birthdays and hospital appointments. These calendars could be used with family members and carers.

Annual calendars produced as gifts or for sale can be created with help from the entire group at different times. For example, computer-confident people could adapt a template, keen photographers could take photos of people, activities and artwork created at the group, and the whole group could create artwork or choose images and designs.

> *Kate was keen to inform families about the week's activities at the day centre. She found a Microsoft Word template that showed a month at a time and was able to add details of outings and events easily. Instead of completing the calendars in the back office, she spent five minutes every Friday and Monday going over the weekly plan with the members of the day centre. She took the laptop to wherever her clients were and adapted each calendar to the activities relevant to that individual.*

### Why use IT?

- There are easily adaptable templates available.
- The same template can be used again and again.
- It is a simple matter to change and update a calendar.
- Calendars can be easily customised for individuals.

## How long will this activity take?

If you are doing this activity with a group it could take many months. If you are planning to sell the next year's calendar or give it to friends of people in the group, remember that it will need to be ready by mid November, and earlier if you want to have it professionally printed.

On the other hand, creating a calendar for the next month's activities may only take an hour or so.

## What will you need?

The equipment you need will vary slightly depending on the type of calendar you plan to produce.

*Essential:*

Computer

Calendar template

Time to plan and to work with people

Printer

*Desirable:*

Digital camera

Laminator

## What could go wrong?

Making individualised weekly or monthly calendars for service users is a commitment. Make sure that there is a small team of staff who are happy to update the calendars.

Planning a calendar over a year for sale or distribution in late autumn is also a commitment. If you are using pictures of activities throughout the year you will need to get consent (see the section 'Confidentiality and consent' in Part 1). Be prepared for the fact that people may get ill, die or leave the service before the calendar is produced.

If you are planning to get the calendar commercially printed, investigate the options, costs and the printer's requirements early on.

## Technical tips

There are many templates available online (for example, via Microsoft Word) that will have the correct dates. Some of these templates will be easier to adapt to your needs than others so it is worth spending some time looking at the different options before you begin.

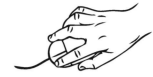

# Greetings cards

Cards are very personal items: they can be made for someone within the group or for families and friends outside the group. They can be made for any occasion: birthday, get well soon, thank you.

Many computer programs provide templates for cards. A template gives an outline of the card that can then be adapted. You can also produce 'e-cards' to send to people with email addresses.

## Who is it useful for?

People with a whole range of abilities can engage in this activity.

- People who are happy using a computer can choose a style template, type in their own message and choose pictures to illustrate the card.

- People who have less ability or confidence can work in a group and contribute by suggesting text, designs or colours, or choose pictures.

- People who do not seem interested in activities centred around the computer can still be part of the group. Incomplete cards can be printed off and decorated by hand.

Groups can work together to create a card for a group member or member of staff. This activity also works well one to one if someone wishes to create a special card for a family member or friend.

> *Sangeeta and her family were celebrating Diwali. This meant that Sangeeta didn't attend the day centre for a week. Her friends there were worried about her absence. When the activities co-ordinator, Mick, tried to explain, Edna and Ethel didn't understand. Mick went online and searched for some appropriate information about Diwali to show to Edna and Ethel. They loved the pictures of candles and lights. Mick saved some of the pictures they found.*
>
> *Edna and Ethel wanted their friend to know they were missing her. Mick found a template of a birthday card that he had used before. He deleted the picture of a birthday cake and the text and then worked with Edna and Ethel to create a 'Happy Diwali' card for Sangeeta. Edna and Ethel added the pictures they had found and typed in a special greeting for Sangeeta.*

### Why use IT?

- There are special programs that are designed to make cards.
- Templates available online can help you too.
- Cards can be saved and used again.
- Multiple copies can be printed.

### How long will this activity take?

Creating a greetings card can be a short activity that produces something to hold quickly. If you are well prepared, making a card can take just half an hour.

### What will you need?

Computer with a reasonable size screen

Either specialist card-making software or word-processing software such as Word

Good colour printer – the better the printer the more accurate the colours will be

Access to the internet for card templates and images

Any specialist equipment that people might need (see the section 'Special equipment' in Part 1)

### What could go wrong?

Know the people you are working with. There is nothing wrong with someone making a card for a friend or relative who has died, but presenting this to another family member may cause distress.

Colour printing can be expensive. Think about the amount of block colour you are printing. Investigate options with more white space and printing on coloured paper or card.

Online services (such as those offering e-cards) mostly require you to register with them. This usually means giving them a valid email address and creating a user name and password. Services that are free online often get their revenue from advertising. Therefore it might be worth setting up a different email address to use when registering for this type of service. That way, any promotional emails will go to this new address rather than the group email address that you use for correspondence.

Routledge
Taylor & Francis Group

### Technical tips

If you think your group will want to make lots of cards, it might be worth investing in some specialist software. Searching online for 'greeting cards software' will give you some ideas.

If you are working with people who want to email friends or relatives, search for e-cards. There are various websites that allow you to choose a pre-designed card, add your message and then email it.

Standard word-processing software, such as Microsoft Word, often has templates that you can work with. Newer versions of Word allow you to access these templates when you create a new document. If your version does not have this option, you can search online for 'Microsoft Office templates', which you can download to your computer and use again and again.

Be aware that some of the templates that are available are for documents designed as a single sheet of paper to be folded into four. This means that the 'front page' quarter has the text upside down.

Practise using templates and designing cards before you try this with the people you work with.

# Other things to take home

Your imagination is the only limit to using the computer to create things for people to take home. Examples include:

- bookmarks
- placemats or coasters
- photo albums
- stickers
- certificates
- invitations.

### Who is it useful for?

This will probably be an ad hoc activity as part of a wider project around an event or art activity. This sort of work is perfect for doing with individuals, but it is also suitable for small groups. Each person can take a turn customising a template. It can also be combined with traditional art and craft activities, for example creating a black and white template for bookmarks, printing them out and giving them to people to paint or decorate.

*Christmas was getting close at the Layer Street peer support group for younger people with dementia. They were planning a party and had agreed on a Hawaiian theme. While the baking group were planning menus, the computer group thought that they could contribute too. They found a lovely picture on a photo library website and used this as the basis for a variety of objects. First they used MS Word to find a template for an invitation. They removed the image and replaced it with the one they had found and adapted the text. They then used presentation software to create placemats for each person at the party. Each one had the individual's name in the centre. They also created menus for the tables.*

### Why use IT?

Using IT means that once you have an idea you can save it to be used in the future. Your template can be customised for an individual or adapted for a different occasion.

### How long will it take?

The length of time needed for these activities will depend on the complexity of the objects you are making. Preparation is vital. It is a good idea to make the objects in advance yourself before you start working with your group.

Routledge Taylor & Francis Group

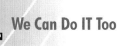

### What will you need?

Computer

Internet access for research and photo libraries

Good-quality colour printer

Lots of printer toner, card and paper

Laminator

Guillotine (for cutting card)

### What could go wrong?

Making things is an ideal opportunity to combine traditional art sessions with computer work. Basic designs can be created on the computer with finishing touches added by the art group.

Some Word templates are complicated so be sure to try them out before you use them with other people.

### Technical tips

Microsoft Word has a variety of ready-made templates that you can investigate.

Many of the examples we have given will involve using card. If you are planning to make items from card, check first that your printer is capable of taking card of different thicknesses.

# Making things to improve the service environment

The environment that people live in can either increase or reduce confusion, communication and memory difficulties. Sensory changes associated with dementia can make the environment difficult to understand. Signalling the difference and function of each room or area can help people understand where they are or locate their room or the bathroom.

It can be difficult for people to recognise the specific features of objects, leading to confusion about how to use them: for example, finding a door handle or turning a basin tap in the right direction. Giving people the opportunity to produce items such as information signs, labels or menus enables them to contribute to their homes, allowing personal 'ownership' and attributing recognisable value to individual efforts. Making practical items ensures that symbols and signs are understood by residents, who are more likely to remember or recognise what they mean.

# Signs

We see signs and symbols all around us, in our homes, in shops, streets and roads. People's ability to understand them often far outlives their ability to make sense of written words (see examples in Part 3) and varies significantly from one person to another.

Encouraging people to become involved in making their own signs and notices gives them the opportunity to choose what they like and what they understand best. Signs can:

- increase understanding of the environment
- encourage independence
- promote choice
- encourage shared understanding.

## Who is it useful for?

This activity is particularly useful for people living in residential homes, although making signs to highlight particular rooms or activities may also promote independence for people living in their own homes.

Routledge
Taylor & Francis Group

The activity is suitable for individuals or groups. The most able participants will be able to identify what they would like to include in the project. They will be able to type into a search engine with only occasional prompting to search for images and copy and paste them into a text box.

Some people will be able to type simple words with support and select from a choice of symbols, whereas others will be able to make a choice from a small range of pictures and symbols and help place the signs in position in the environment.

> *Moira was living independently at home. She had meals delivered to her. One day Moira rang her daughter in a panic saying that she had opened the cutlery drawer and could not find a knife anywhere. Moira could not understand this and had become very agitated and upset. Her daughter called round to help her and when she looked in the drawer there were many knives, forks and spoons there. Moira had visual perceptual difficulties and had begun to have difficulties understanding everyday objects in her environment. As soon as Moira was encouraged to reach into the drawer and touch the items she recognised the cutlery straight away.*

## Why use IT?

- It is easy to search for a choice of symbols and pictures.
- Signs produced can be easily duplicated to use in more than one environment.
- The size of pictures can easily be changed.
- Printed signs are clearer and can be laminated and wiped down.

## How long will this activity take?

Individual signs can be produced in a 30-minute session. Producing signage for a number of rooms or occasions should be an activity taking several weeks, as making too many symbols and pictures in one long activity session may be confusing for participants.

## What will you need?

*Essential:*

PC or laptop

Internet connection

Good-quality printer

Some white and coloured card

*Desirable:*

Laminator

## What could go wrong?

People may struggle to find a symbol that they understand or to come to a consensus about what to select.

## Technical tips

Open a text box and paste the chosen picture into it. It will then be much easier to move around the page.

Choose high contrast colours, for example black on yellow, to increase visibility.

Consider using photographs rather than symbols. We have found that people with dementia are happier with photographs than highly stylised images.

When using a laminator, check the manufacturer's instructions carefully, especially with reference to the heat settings, as it is possible to 'melt' the laminating sheets or lose valuable work in the laminator.

  Routledge
Taylor & Francis Group

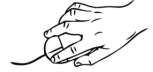

# Menus

People with dementia often have difficulty with eating and drinking. They may 'forget' how to eat and drink or how to use cutlery, or their tastes may have radically altered. It is important to optimise enjoyment of eating and drinking and continue to offer appropriate choices as far as possible.

People may find it easier to choose what they want to eat when shown the selection of real food on a plate. However, this may not always be an option. Having photographs of meals on the menu as they are to be presented has been shown to be an effective way to enable people to make an informed choice about food and drink. Photographic menus may:

- support people's ability to make a choice
- make choices transparent
- make mealtimes more enjoyable
- involve service users in creating their environment.

## Who is it useful for?

This activity is particularly useful for residential settings, although photographic choices could be useful for individuals in any environment.

The activity involves many different processes and is suitable for both individuals and groups during the various stages.

Some people will be confident using a digital camera independently and may just need help with setting up to take photographs of food. The advantage of digital photography is that you can take several photographs of the same subject and discard the ones that are not needed. Downloading photographs to the computer is more challenging and most people will need considerable help with this unless they have had previous experience.

Some people will enjoy typing labels on to the meal pictures and printing and laminating them. They may need help with using the keyboard and placing text in the chosen position.

People who require more assistance will still enjoy looking at the pictures and identifying them. It is useful to have a mixed group of abilities in order to research whether people recognise the meals depicted in the photographs.

## Why use IT?

Digital photography is an essential tool for obtaining clear illustrations that can be produced in varying sizes with text easily added as required.

## How long will this activity take?

Producing photographic menus involves a number of stages that will take place over several weeks or months. As menus change, photographs will need to be regularly updated, so this is an ongoing project. Weekly menus tend to rotate over several weeks and photographs of all the savoury and sweet options need to be taken. This task can be undertaken by one individual or rotated around a group of people.

A group can then be formed to work on a template and produce photographs. Once a template has been agreed and established, individual photographs can be easily replaced with new ones as menu options change.

For best effect, the day's options need to be available at every table so that each individual can select their choice of meal. These often become a talking point while people wait in the dining room for meals to be served.

## What will you need?

*Essential:*

Digital camera

Printer

Laminator

Good-quality paper

A method of displaying the photographs on each table

*Desirable:*

PC or laptop to resize, save photographs and add text

## What could go wrong?

Although extremely worthwhile, this project is time-consuming and requires commitment to keep it going when photographs need to be replaced.

## Technical tips

Make sure you have plenty of coloured ink and a good-quality printer, and that food is presented clearly on plain plates against a contrasting background so that it is easily recognisable.

 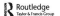

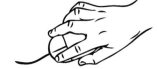

# Newsletters

Newsletters are a great way of bringing everyone involved with a service together. They are useful for:

- keeping in touch with family or friends who may not have much contact with the service
- reminding staff and service users about activities
- publicising future events
- recording achievements
- proving the worth of your service to management or funders.

## Who is it useful for?

Many services produce newsletters, but they are often produced by staff or volunteers without input from service users. If you have introduced computer work into your service, creating a newsletter is an ideal way of bringing all the work together. Everyone in the service can be involved in some way. For example, key members of staff could work with members of the computer or media group to plan, design and produce the newsletter. Others can be involved in a variety of ways, for example:

- being interviewed or photographed
- being involved in design decisions
- taking photographs.

*Rodney was a new member of staff and keen to make his mark. He quickly took part in all the computer-related activities at the day centre. Jan put him in charge of the newsletter project with an 'editorial board' of people with dementia and two other key members of staff. They found a template of a two-page newsletter in columns. They agreed on regular features including 'what's happening next month', a regular feature on one of the members of staff, and reports of outings or activities.*

*Throughout the month Rodney took every opportunity to collect information and ask people to take photographs for the newsletter. However, he also ensured that the computer group dedicated two sessions a month to the newsletter production. After a couple of issues were distributed to families and friends, Sangeeta's grandson contacted Rodney. He was doing a media course at the local college and thought he could help ...*

### Why use IT?

Before computers became commonplace it was very difficult to produce newsletters. A computer makes the process easy. Once a template has been chosen, it can be adapted each time for new text and images.

Newsletters produced electronically can be printed or sent by email.

### How long will this activity take?

This will depend on how long the newsletter is and how many people are involved. It is a good idea to make sure that some dedicated staff time and contact time with the service users is set aside regularly. Including a regular feature on different members of the service will need time.

### What will you need?

Computer with suitable software

Member of staff willing to take the lead

Other staff and people with dementia who are interested

Support from management

Printer – and photocopier for creating multiple copies

Digital camera

Method for distributing the newsletter – via post or email to relatives and other interested people

### What could go wrong?

It is easy to have enthusiasm for starting a newsletter, but it is a commitment. Make sure that there is wide support among staff, management, people with dementia and their families and carers.

Don't be too ambitious – creating a newsletter every month is a big commitment as it is a time-consuming activity. Maybe quarterly would be more appropriate.

If you are featuring service users be sure to obtain consent to use their name or photograph (see the section 'Confidentiality and consent' in Part 1).

### Technical tips

Take some time to get the right template. We have given you an example of how it could look in Part 3. Text in columns is easier to read, but think about your audience. Do you need to make the text bigger than usual for a newsletter?

 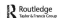

Also consider how you will be reproducing and distributing the newsletter. If you need to make a large number of photocopies of it do not use colour unless you have a colour copier and the budget to pay for the copies.

If you want to email the newsletter consider creating a PDF file. A PDF file preserves the formatting of your original document.

# Helping with conversations

People who have been diagnosed with dementia often have some form of communication difficulty. They may experience specific problems with understanding language, especially long, complex instructions or conversations between several people.

When someone acquires a communication difficulty as an adult they do not lose all their understanding of the world and their experiences. They may have a good understanding of 'social' rules such looking at people who are talking to them, showing interest in what they are saying and responding with appropriate smiles or facial expression. The ability to follow these social rules can sometimes mask difficulties with understanding language. It may be that they can understand actions but not the specific words people are saying. They may realise that someone has asked a question by the tone of their voice but not precisely what that question is. It may be that they have understood part of what was being said but have not been able to follow the whole conversation. They may only be able to respond to part of a question or instruction.

Some people have difficulties forming words or sentences. We have all experienced frustration when the word we want is on the 'tip of our tongue'. Sometimes these expressive difficulties can be very significant, with people being unable to name even close family or friends, familiar places or names of common objects or foods. They may even confuse the words 'yes' and 'no'. Making choices, asking people even simple questions or just trying to have a chat can be really difficult.

It is important to encourage people with communication difficulties to be as independent as possible and to use as many methods of getting a message across as they can. Getting together in groups with friends or family or with other people who are experiencing communication difficulties is an important way of using new skills and methods of communicating and also provides an opportunity to discuss specific problems and find out how other people manage.

Routledge
Taylor & Francis Group

# Aided topic discussion for people with communication difficulties

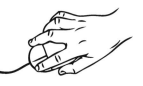

People who experience communication difficulties may benefit from having information presented in a variety of different ways. They may be able to use 'communication ramps' such as maps, pictures, diaries and calendars more effectively than words (Parr *et al*, 2004). Even when people's language is intact these items can be good memory aids.

> *Marcus had difficulty understanding complex language and was experiencing very severe word finding difficulties, especially with names of places and people.*
>
> *Prior to these difficulties Marcus had been an active member of his local council and found that some of his previous colleagues were not very understanding about his communication difficulties and were embarrassed when they met him out in the town centre. He had very few opportunities to socialise.*
>
> *Marcus continued to enjoy family holidays and could use maps and atlases well. He began to attend a group run by the local speech and language therapy service. The group used 'communication ramps' such as objects, newspapers, maps, photographs and pictures to optimise communication. Marcus felt that this was a group of people who could understand the frustrations and isolation he was experiencing. He began to use his abilities with maps and pictures to have conversations with other people in the group.*
>
> *Marcus and his wife became friendly with another couple who attended the group and they often planned trips together. As a consequence Marcus was less frustrated and was more relaxed about joining in conversations.*

Topic discussion groups aim to:

- support people with communication needs
- give all group members an equal chance to express themselves
- support those with memory difficulties in engaging in meaningful discussion.

## Who is it useful for?

Aided topic discussion is useful for anyone who is experiencing communication difficulties. Using a variety of different media can help to engage people who are experiencing memory difficulties as well. A multisensory approach taps into all of a person's residual abilities.

Topic discussion can be either an individual or a group activity, although it is particularly useful for encouraging group conversations and ensuring that all group members have an opportunity to participate. Some groups may run quite independently and only need setting up. Supplying the materials for discussion and being on hand to make the refreshments and provide technical support when using the equipment may be all that is needed.

If people are experiencing problems with communication and turn taking, and if the group is made up of people with a range of abilities, you will need a more rigid structure, introducing the topic yourself and giving each group member an opportunity to contribute as well as setting up any technical equipment. It may be possible for individuals to bring in their own objects, pictures and other materials from home, but they could need prompting to describe their interests with questions from the group.

Some people who have severe communication and memory difficulties may rely heavily on your support. They may be able to relate better to objects and printed pictures than to words and internet searches.

Sometimes using a computer can be a good way of preparing for the group. If you are aware of an interest, for example a particular artist or musician, then searching for information and materials to stimulate discussion can be done before the group session.

*Michael was very keen on horse racing. He had significant word-finding and memory difficulties. During a discussion about sport Michael remembered that he had been to a racecourse when he was a child. He was particularly animated and could point out that the racecourse was in the south of England, although he could not remember the name of it. A quick search on the internet brought up a list of racecourses in southern England and Michael was able to choose the one he meant from a list. It was then possible to find photographs of the racecourse for the group to look at.*

*Linda was invited to attend a discussion group. She found it difficult to relax in a group setting and had problems initiating any communication. A meeting with Linda and her husband was arranged a few days before the group was due to meet for the first time and Linda's husband told us that she had a real interest in jazz music. A musical theme was used for the first meeting and it was possible to prepare for this by searching for and printing some information and pictures to help Linda feel included. Linda and the other group members each brought in a favourite piece of music and everyone contributed to the group and enjoyed discovering some mutual interests as well as being introduced to new musical styles.*

Routledge
Taylor & Francis Group

### Why use IT?

Using a computer and digital photography can help provide some stimulating and useful material instantly. For example, if someone has brought up a topic and no magazines or objects are available to illustrate it, a quick web search can often provide pictures, maps and other visual materials.

### How long will this activity take?

A group discussion can be 'as long as a piece of string'! However, meaningful discussions with people who are experiencing communication difficulties can be held in a group lasting about an hour.

### What will you need?

*Essential:*

Some planning around a chosen topic (after the initial session the group can decide on the following sessions)

Interesting objects that reflect a topic: for example, the topic 'holidays' might include maps, atlases, brochures, swimwear, sun block, train tickets

Computer with large monitor

Internet connection

Two people to run a group

*Desirable:*

CD/MP3 player and music reflecting the chosen topic

A means of recording the group: digital camera, voice recording equipment

### What could go wrong?

Finding a topic that everyone wants to contribute to might be difficult.

Some group members may dominate the discussion and you will need skill to ensure everyone is included. Some people will find it difficult to initiate and will need support to formulate questions.

### Technical tips

Have your internet connection and search engine open so that you can search quickly. It is difficult for people with communication and memory difficulties to sustain their attention while somebody is turning on a computer.

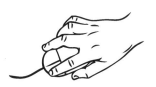

# Reminiscence

Reminiscence is an established technique used with people with dementia. It involves the discussion of past activities, events and experiences. Objects, photographs and music are often used to encourage people with dementia to talk about their past.

## Who is it useful for?

Reminiscence can be done individually or in groups. Reminiscence groups typically involve meetings in which participants are encouraged to talk about past events at least once a week. However, reminiscence work can be done on an ad hoc basis whenever seems appropriate.

As people are encouraged to talk, the computer is used as a tool to produce prompts for further discussion.

> *Sergio wasn't interested in computer work and found it difficult to join in with general reminiscence discussions with others at the day centre. He came originally from Chile and did not share many of the memories of childhoods in England. Staff found it difficult to get him to talk about his background. One day Stephanie was using the website YouTube to find music for Annie to sing to. She asked Sergio if he had any requests. He mentioned a name that meant nothing to her. Luckily, YouTube recognised the Spanish opera singer. The music was beautiful – Annie enjoyed it – and Sergio started to talk a little about his past.*

## Why use IT?

Using IT, and in particular the internet, can be very useful for reminiscence. By searching the internet, you can:

- ensure that reminiscence sessions are tailored to the people you are working with
- obtain a variety of prompts, including text, sound, images and video
- allow the people reminiscing to guide the session by having the flexibility to go off on tangents.

## How long will this activity take?

Individual reminiscence sessions will probably not last much more than 60 minutes. However, it is a good idea to do some preparatory work and have some standby websites saved as favourites or bookmarks that you know will be useful. Alternatively, you could print out some pictures beforehand so that people have something to start with and are not focused entirely on the screen.

 Routledge
Taylor & Francis Group

## What will you need?

Computer with internet access

Printer to print out anything of interest that you find

Projector if working with groups so that everyone can see the screen easily

Speakers if you are going to be retrieving sound

Time to plan some searches

## What could go wrong?

The internet is a vast resource that is not policed in any way. When using search engines you need to be careful. For example:

- Choose your words carefully. Many everyday words may have a double meaning with the result that you may retrieve pornography or other websites you were not expecting!

- Many websites are full of words and not particularly stimulating or engaging. Try searching just for images at first.

- Some people may have events in their past that they do not want to remember or that bring up upsetting issues. This is not always a bad thing, but you need to be prepared.

## Technical tips

The internet is a vast source of information, video clips and images. When you have found something of interest it is worth keeping it. There are two ways to do this:

1. Use the bookmarking or favourites system on your internet browser software. This allows you to save the addresses of useful websites that you want to revisit. You can go directly to a particular website from the list you create without having to search for it again.

2. Save images or text to individual folders on the computer. These could be created for each person you work with or you could have a general folder for reminiscence work with the whole group.

Search engines such as Google allow you to search specifically for images or maps.

# Family trees

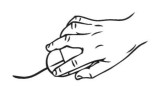

People with memory difficulties are at risk of losing their sense of identity. They may find it difficult to name, or even recognise, previously familiar friends or close family members. This can be extremely distressing for both the person and for those who care for them. Family and friends may be spread over a wide geographical area and some may even have emigrated. New grandchildren or great grandchildren may be entering the family and relationships may be being formed or broken.

The aims of making a family tree are to:

- support memory
- help reduce individual frustration
- remind people about how they relate to past and present family members.

## Who is it useful for?

This activity is particularly useful for those people who are beginning to find it difficult to remember family names and recognise extended family members. Making a family tree is most suitable as an individual activity. However, some aspects of this activity can be explored as a 'family' topic in a discussion group.

The most confident participants will be able to name their immediate relatives and enter text independently on to a template. They may be able to copy and paste photographs to illustrate their family tree or add additional family information.

People who are inexperienced in using IT can still participate by providing stories and information about their relatives. It would be nice to include some historical anecdotes and these could be recorded as text with support or using a recordable compact disc, digital voice recorder or cassette tapes.

People who need full assistance may be able to tell you who is in their photographs, or their relationship with people, or be able to confirm the names of relatives. They could possibly tell you interesting information about family members such as schools attended and places lived in or visited, and give you key words that could be used to search the internet for appropriate information. The end product will be a stimulating resource to use as part of other activities.

*Gerald had significant memory difficulties. He was living at home but his wife was finding it extremely difficult to manage and had made the decision that Gerald needed to be cared for in a residential setting. While Gerald was still at home she worked with him to produce a simple family tree covering his parents, brothers*

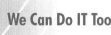

and sisters, children and grandchildren. She used a separate page for each generation as Gerald found this less confusing.

Gerald really enjoyed looking at old family photographs and recalled some family tales that his wife had forgotten. She typed these out and included them in the family tree. Staff at his new home loved looking at Gerald's family tree and he enjoyed talking about incidents that had been recorded as well as remembering a few more that his wife was able to use to update his book.

## Why use IT?

Family trees can be very complex and may include step-relationships or several marriages or partnerships. Using a computer gives valuable flexibility and allows visual information to be presented in a variety of ways to suit individual needs and abilities. Word-processing software will let you add or update information easily and you can include photos, pictures and other information. Work can be revisited and updated at any time.

## How long will this activity take?

Making a family tree will inevitably involve some preparation and discussion with family members in order to obtain accurate information. It is good, however, to start by working with the participant to find out from them what they can remember. Any gaps can then be filled by talking to relatives or friends. Family trees can be a simple one-page record of immediate family (see the example in Part 3) or can span many generations.

The time this will take depends on how much information is included. The most important aspect is to focus on each session and encourage participants to recall treasured events and memories. The finished piece of work can then be used as a daily memory aid, included in life history books or used in topic discussion groups.

It may be possible to include friends as well as relatives in a family tree.

## What will you need?

*Essential:*

Family names and information

Computer with word-processing software

Printer

*Desirable:*

Photographs

Scanner so that original photographs do not have to be used

File or folder with plastic sleeves for the finished project

## What could go wrong?

It can take time for families to provide the information requested.

Some information may bring back painful memories and some family members may have left the family and no longer be in contact.

People may have little or no recollection of some of their relatives. A decision needs to be made in all cases about whom to include.

## Technical tips

Save work frequently to avoid losing it. Check that the font and style you choose are suitable for each person. It may be a good idea to differentiate the information in some way, for example having all females in one colour and males in another or choosing a different font or colour to mark the different generations.

There are a number of internet sites (that require subscription) that can help when searching for information such as electoral registers. However, many of these are complicated to use, so investigate them before you start using them with people with dementia.

 Routledge
Taylor & Francis Group

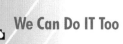

# Communicating with friends and family

There are many ways of communicating with friends and family using IT. We will discuss email, voice over the internet (eg Skype) and social networking.

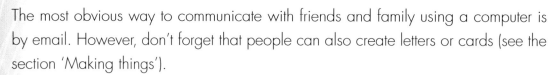

## Email

The most obvious way to communicate with friends and family using a computer is by email. However, don't forget that people can also create letters or cards (see the section 'Making things').

### Who is it useful for?

If you are working with a group, it is a good idea to have one group email address. Try getting in contact with other groups who may be able to email your group.

Keeping in contact with family and friends will often naturally be an individual activity. People who can use the keyboard will benefit most from this activity, but you can assist people to send photographs or digital artwork.

> *All the members of the computer club have heard of email. They are interested to see how it works. John, the activities co-ordinator, has created a Googlemail account for the whole group. They use it to communicate with another computer club they have heard about at a day centre on the other side of the country. Every Thursday they log into the account. They reply to the previous email and tell the other group about what they have been doing.*

### Why use IT?

Email is a very easy way to communicate. Advantages for people with memory problems are:

- The email system will store copies of all emails sent, so that they can be easily referred back to.

- Many people will reply and keep the original text in the system.

- Most systems include an address book, so people do not need to remember addresses.

- People can communicate with friends and family around the world.

- Photos can easily be included.

## How long will it take?

Reading and sending email messages will only take a few minutes. Try to make it a regular activity.

## What will you need?

Computer with internet access

A method of keeping email usernames and passwords safe

Printer to print out messages that can be taken home

## What could go wrong?

One of the most difficult things to remember is passwords. If people have individual email accounts, keep a list of usernames and passwords.

Make sure that the person your client is communicating with is willing and able to reply, as it can be a little upsetting to send an email and not receive a reply. If this happens it might be an idea to check the email address.

Confidentiality is important: make sure everyone understands that staff are assisting with email and consequently communication is not completely confidential.

All email addresses are subject to spam, that is, unsolicited email. It is worth taking a bit of time to regularly check email accounts to delete spam before people access them.

## Technical tips

There are many different ways of accessing email. Your internet service provider (ISP) will provide you with an address but you can also get web-only email from services such as Yahoo and Google.

  Routledge
Taylor & Francis Group

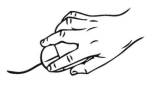

# Voice over the internet (eg Skype)

Skype is the best-known software that allows people to talk to each other via the computer rather than the telephone. The software is free, but will have to be downloaded from the Skype website and you may be asked to buy some credit.

## Who is it useful for?

Using Skype in a dementia care setting is probably most useful for a group communicating with another group that meets in a different setting, although individual calls to friends and relations would also be possible. Once you have set up the computer and internet connection at your service, you may be approached by the family or friends of people with dementia who have a relation somewhere abroad who would like to communicate with them via Skype.

*Annie had recently had to move into residential care after her husband and main carer died. She had been an active member of the computer club and was reluctant to lose contact with her friends. Sarah promised that they would keep in contact. Annie's granddaughter set up a computer, webcam and Skype in Annie's room at the nursing home and Sarah did the same at the day centre. They agreed on a time when Annie's granddaughter would be there to help her and the computer club group would be meeting at the day centre, so they could all talk together.*

## Why use IT?

The advantages of Skype over the telephone are:

- Skype calls to other Skype users are 'free', that is, there are no additional charges. However, both parties have to be online.

- You can use a webcam, which means that you can see the other person as well as hearing their voice.

You can use your Skype account to ring telephone numbers but this service will incur a cost.

## How long will this activity take?

Skype will take some time to set up, but once you are connected it is like speaking to someone on the telephone. However, you will need to coordinate with the other person or group to ensure that everyone is online at the same time.

## What will you need?

Computer with an internet connection

Skype software and account

Microphone and speakers, or a headset for private calls

Someone to talk to who has Skype set up and the time and ability to talk at the moment you want them to.

## What could go wrong?

Only you will be able to tell if this facility is appropriate for your setting. Providing people with the means to make private phone calls may not be appropriate. However, if your group likes to talk to other groups this is a cheap and interesting way to do so. The biggest problem (as with email) is that you need to be in contact with a like-minded group that meets at the same time as yours.

People with hearing problems may have more problems with Skype than with a telephone.

## Technical tips

Make sure that you set up Skype properly and in particular check the privacy settings. Unless you specify otherwise, your Skype name will appear to other Skype users every time you are online and you may get unwanted calls.

Test and check the positioning of your webcam so that the whole group is visible. Also check the sensitivity of the microphone, as you want everyone in the group to be able to contribute.

Routledge
Taylor & Francis Group

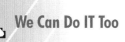 

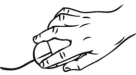

# Social networking and discussion forums

Social networking is a recent trend. You will have heard of and probably used sites such as Facebook, MySpace and Twitter. Social networking sites link people together in a variety of ways. Many charity and other special interest sites will have discussion groups that allow people to post messages to others about different topics.

## Who is it useful for?

Most of these sites are very much focused on the individual. However, some of your group members may have, or may be encouraged to have, accounts with Facebook or other social networking accounts. Depending on the focus of your group, they may want to contribute to discussions that you find on the web, for example the Alzheimer's Society's Talking Point forum.

> *Karim was a regular Facebook user since his daughter suggested he join. He was also a contributor to Alzheimer's Talking Point. However, his computer at home had broken and it was a few months since he had been online. The main reason for him agreeing to attend the day centre was that he had been told he could use the computer.*
>
> *Karim had a few problems with the day centre computer. It was newer than his and the icons were in different places. He also had problems remembering his passwords. But Jan sat down with him and went through everything. She wrote down the sequence of actions needed to get on to Facebook and then worked with Karim to remember his password.*

## Why use IT?

This type of activity is only available through the internet. Some members of your group may have no idea or concept of social networking or online discussions, but others will have used these sites and will be grateful for your support in enabling them to continue this hobby. Many younger people live much of their lives through these sites and could not imagine being without them. Many charities and interest groups have Facebook pages to promote their work and engage with supporters.

## How long will it take?

Some people spend many hours on Facebook communicating with friends. There are also online games that can be played through many of these sites.

## What will you need?

Computer with internet access

A way of storing people's passwords securely

## What could go wrong?

Privacy on the internet is a big concern, and many people do not realise who might be able to see the information they are posting. Each website will have a different way of changing who can see different bits of information. Look for something called 'privacy settings' or 'security'.

Only you can decide if an internet café style service of supporting people to access their private email and social networking sites via your computers is appropriate.

## Technical tips

Facebook and other sites are quite complex. If you are supporting people to use such facilities it would be worth your while to investigate all the options.

One of the main reasons for people using Facebook and other social networking sites is to share photographs. People may need support to transfer the pictures from their personal cameras to Facebook. The easiest way is to suggest they ask a high street photo-processing shop to put the photos on to a CD.

 Routledge Taylor & Francis Group

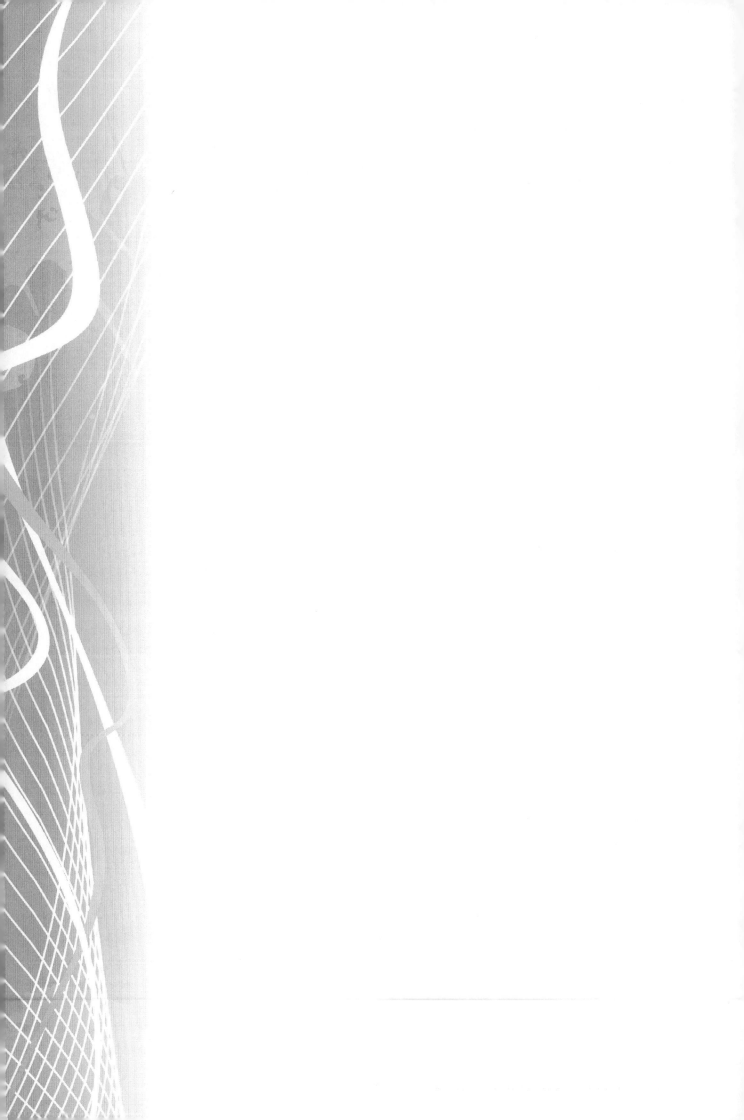

# Helping with planning

Planning can take many forms. In this section we talk about using IT as a tool to help include people with dementia in two types of planning: personal advance care planning and more general planning of service development.

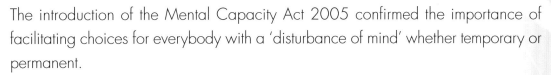

## Personal planning

The introduction of the Mental Capacity Act 2005 confirmed the importance of facilitating choices for everybody with a 'disturbance of mind' whether temporary or permanent.

Although this is a sensitive subject to approach, it is important at the diagnosis of a mental illness to discuss a person's future and especially their wishes regarding social and medical care. Decisions around these issues can be difficult and emotional, but if personal preferences are not recorded it is left to family and professionals to make decisions as the need arises.

It is, of course, possible for someone to name trusted family or friends as appointees to make social or medical decisions for them should they ever lack the capacity to do so, and information regarding this can be found on the website of the Office of the Public Guardian. More information regarding the Mental Capacity Act can be found on the website of the Department of Constitutional Affairs. (See the References for addresses.)

The aims of personal planning are to:

- ensure the person's wishes are understood by everyone
- influence their future social and/or medical care
- relieve family members of doubt and concern should they be called on to give their opinion.

### Who is it useful for?

Many people want to plan for their future social and medical care, and the process of planning future care should begin as early as possible. This is a time when making changes such as moving house or appointing a power of attorney could enable

Routledge
Taylor & Francis Group

future independence and reduce reliance on outside agencies for care until much later on. For example, moving house at a late stage in life can be very disorientating for a person with significant memory difficulties, and such an important change can exacerbate problems with daily living tasks such as shopping and cooking.

Planning future care needs to be done on an individual basis with someone who is impartial. It is an emotive subject and needs to be sensitively handled.

At initial diagnosis a person may have initiated the process of formulating and writing plans for the future. They may need help with accessing pro-formas online or advice about the best format for their plans. If they wish to use word processing they may need help using the functions of the software.

A pro-forma that prompts the user, through questions, to supply the information that is required can be helpful. Wishes can be recorded in writing or by voice recording or typing.

Even someone who has significant memory difficulties may be able to express their opinions and wishes for the future. It may be useful to print photographs and pictures of choices and determine through dialogue what someone's preferences are.

> *Philip had been diagnosed with a progressive physical illness as well as showing the early signs of dementia. His ability to swallow was deteriorating and he was given some information about enteral feeding alternatives. Philip was against the idea of being fed through a tube and completed an 'advance decision to refuse treatment' using a form that he had downloaded from the internet.*
>
> *Several months later Philip was admitted to hospital with a broken hip. His swallowing had deteriorated and he was finding it uncomfortable to eat. Despite his earlier decision, Philip realised that his physical condition was deteriorating far faster than his memory and decided that he would like a feeding tube to prevent him from losing weight and possibly getting chest infections or pneumonia.*

## Why use IT?

It is important that information regarding people's wishes and plans is clearly presented and safely stored. A number of people or agencies may need copies, and using a document that has been word-processed, dated, printed and signed ensures that it is legible. If safely stored, documents can be revisited and updated as long as they are reprinted, dated and signed appropriately.

## How long will this activity take?

Planning future care will take many weeks and needs to be revisited as often as a person would like. The plans may change in the light of new information and feelings and are not to be thought of as unalterable. We all make different decisions or change our minds as circumstances change and our knowledge increases.

## What will you need?

*Essential:*

An experienced person who is impartial but who understands the process

Knowledge of legal issues and obligations

Personal computer or laptop

Printer

Witnesses as necessary

Secure storage

*Desirable:*

A pro-forma that directs you to include essential information – this may increase the validity of the document if it is used as evidence of a person's wishes, should they lack the capacity to make a particular decision

An option to record someone's decisions about future care using voice-recording equipment

## What could go wrong?

You may doubt that the participant has the capacity to make complex decisions or be concerned that they appear to be making foolish choices. You may feel it is difficult to remain impartial if you believe that the plans being made are wrong or ones that you would not choose yourself. You may find that family or friends do not agree with the plans that have been made and think that their relative is no longer able to make decisions.

The Mental Capacity Act has five main principles, the third of which states 'A person is not to be treated as unable to make a decision merely because he makes an unwise decision' (Mental Capacity Act 2005, Part 1).

There are clear principles and procedures to follow that should lead to a decision about whether someone lacks capacity to make a particular decision. Someone who lacks capacity cannot do one or more of the following:

  Routledge
Taylor & Francis Group

- understand information given to them
- retain information long enough to make a decision
- weigh up the information available to make a decision
- communicate their decision.

You may want to seek advice from an experienced professional. However, it is everyone's responsibility to follow the guidance and record decisions about capacity carefully. It may be that family members do not always have their relative's best interests at heart.

## Technical tips

If planning involves issues of medical treatment it is important that the person making a decision is fully informed. Professional advice should be sought from a general practitioner or health care professional. A useful pro-forma regarding an advance decision to refuse medical treatment can be found on the website of the National Health Service's National End of Life Care Programme (NHS, 2008).

# Planning services – supporting meetings

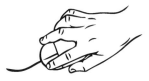

Many groups, including those at day centres and in care homes, have weekly meetings in which all the clients, members or residents meet with the staff to discuss the activities of the group and practical matters such as menus, transport and so on.

### Who is it useful for?

The use of IT to support meetings should be a group activity that includes everyone present. However, it is important to use different people's skills, so assigning tasks that can be rotated around different group members is a good idea, for example typing up notes, taking photos, researching different topics.

> *Margot had always had quarterly meetings at the day centre where people were encouraged to think about the outings for the next quarter. These had always been half-hearted affairs as people seemed keen to agree to any trip suggested. After the computer club started at the centre, she decided to use the computer and projector at the centre meetings. With a little preparation from the computer club members, Margot was able to display pictures of various destinations and attractions to the whole group and observe reactions to the pictures.*

### Why use IT?

Using IT can enhance these meetings. By working with members of the group who like to use IT, the meetings can be even more of a shared experience. Instead of doing the administration for the meeting in the back office, paperwork can be done together with clients or residents.

### How long will it take?

A certain amount of administration will have to be done for these meetings. It is worth taking a bit of extra time to include people in this process.

### What will you need?

Computer

Printer

Possibly a camera and projector

Routledge
Taylor & Francis Group

### What could go wrong?

It is important to try to involve as many clients or residents as possible. Working with just a few who are happy using computers may cause resentment.

### Technical tips

There are various ways in which IT can be used. For example:

- An agenda for the meeting could be typed up with a small group and printed out and distributed.

- The decisions made at the meeting can be recorded with the help of clients or residents.

- The meeting could be photographed or video-recorded to aid people's memories.

- Research into different activities can be carried out using the internet.

- A projector could be used to show images or website pages to the entire group.

# Practical examples

You will find some examples of these projects in the following section. These are intended to give you some ideas about layouts and levels of skill required. It is always important to use layouts, fonts and styles that suit each individual or group, although it may help to make up some templates of your own in advance of projects to reduce the technical difficulties during activities.

Routledge
Taylor & Francis Group

# Part 3 Examples

# How to use this section

This section contains examples of forms and projects that we have introduced in Part 2. We hope that they will give you an idea of how a finished project will look, although, of course, you will probably have some better ideas of your own! Projects and activities are so much better when they are personalised and allow individual creativity.

We have given an idea of the range of skills required for each example and hope that you will see that people of all abilities can be involved in some way. We are sure that in no time you will have found ways to use IT to suit yourself and people with dementia. The most important thing is to enjoy experimenting – and don't forget to 'save' your work as you go, as computers have a habit of freezing or shutting down when you least expect it!

# Invitation letter

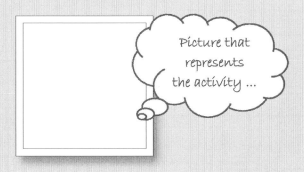

Fairways Community Hospital
24 Coventry Road
Irchester
NN13 1RY
Telephone 02768 435723

Dear

The media group are getting together for 4 sessions of computer activities.
We are meeting at **Newcliffe Community Centre**.

The group begins at **2pm** and ends at **4pm**.
The dates are:       Friday 1st October
                     Friday 8th October
                     Friday 15th October
                     Friday 22nd October

We hope that you can join us and enjoy a drink and a chat as well as
learning more about computers.

I will give you a call nearer the time to see if you are able to come and to
answer any questions.

With best wishes

Jane Smith

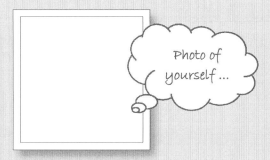

Routledge
Taylor & Francis Group

# Consent form

*Insert name/ logo of organisation.*

*(Insert name of organisation or group)* will use these photographs/this film for *(insert purpose)* purposes. The photographs/film may be viewed by members of the public, families, carers and students.

We will contact you before using the photographs/film for reasons other than the intended purpose.

Photographs/film description:

Purpose of use:

Name of subject _____

Address _____

_____

Telephone number _____

Email _____

I grant permission for *(name of organisation)* to use this photograph/film of me for *(insert purpose)* as described above. I understand that the photographs/film are the property of *(name of organisation)*.

Signed _____

Print _____ Date_____

A copy of this form is to be given to the photograph/film subject.

**To request a copy of the photographs/film or to discuss their use please contact:**
*(Insert name and contact details here)*

_____

_____

# Risk assessment

**Name of assessor:** _____

**Date:** _____  **Review date:** _____

**Describe the hazard:**

*Mark the most appropriate boxes.*

| Possible harm resulting from the hazard | **Minor** | **Serious** | **Moderate** | **Fatal** |
|---|---|---|---|---|
| | | | | |

| Likelihood of harm occurring | **Unlikely** | **Possible** | **Likely** | **Highly likely** |
|---|---|---|---|---|
| | | | | |

**Precautions:**

*The consequences and likelihood of harm should be less following precautions.*

| Possible harm with precautions in place | **Minor** | **Serious** | **Moderate** | **Fatal** |
|---|---|---|---|---|
| | | | | |

| Likelihood of harm with precautions in place | **Unlikely** | **Possible** | **Likely** | **Highly likely** |
|---|---|---|---|---|
| | | | | |

Routledge
Taylor & Francis Group

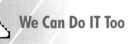 

# Life story book

## Skills

- Narrative about life events
- Selecting pictures
- Naming places and people
- Entering text
- Selecting fonts

- Creating text boxes
- Inserting pictures
- Designing pages
- Searching the internet
- Printing

*This is a sample life story book. The information and pictures contained do not relate to a real person.*

# Life story book for:

# John Smith

# My Name is
# John Smith

I have dementia and sometimes find it difficult to SPEAK, READ or WRITE

This book helps me to tell you a little about myself

R Routledge
Taylor & Francis Group

I was born in Wales, in a town called Aberystwyth

Include maps and personal photographs.

Many people with memory difficulties find they can continue to use maps well.

My Father was an accountant

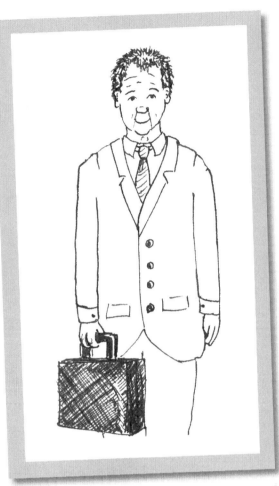

And my Mother was a teacher

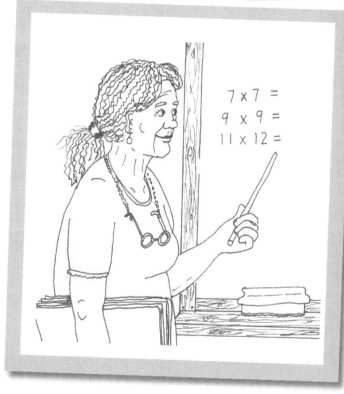

Routledge
Taylor & Francis Group

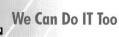

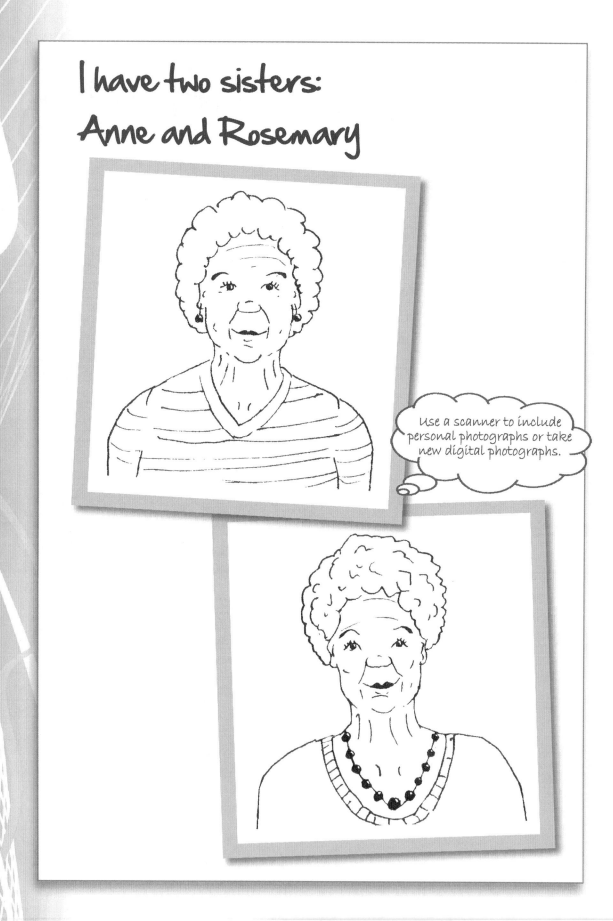

# I have two sisters: Anne and Rosemary

Use a scanner to include personal photographs or take new digital photographs.

I am married to Ruth

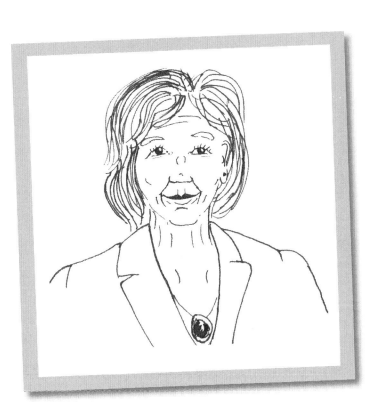

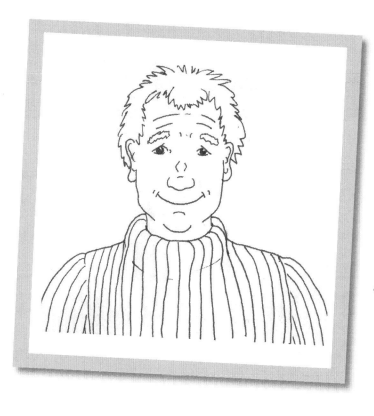

And we have one son called David

Routledge
Taylor & Francis Group

# David is married to Claire

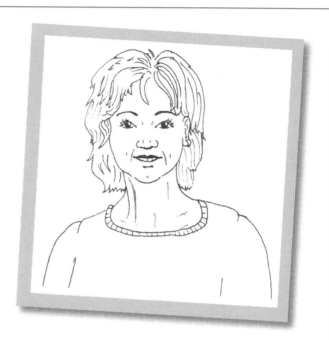

# We have two granddaughters:

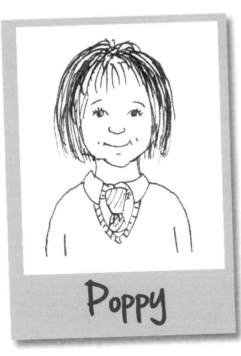

Poppy

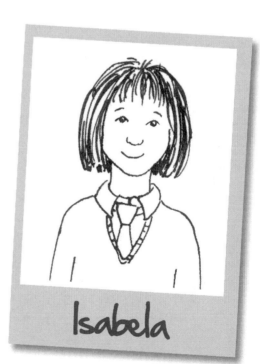

Isabela

Include some scanned drawings done by the children or a favourite poem or anecdote.

I worked as an engineer for a Company called:

**Whates**

Add company information or logo.
You could add favourite anecdotes about work.

Near Radford Semele, Leamington Spa

Where we have lived for 32 years

Routledge
Taylor & Francis Group

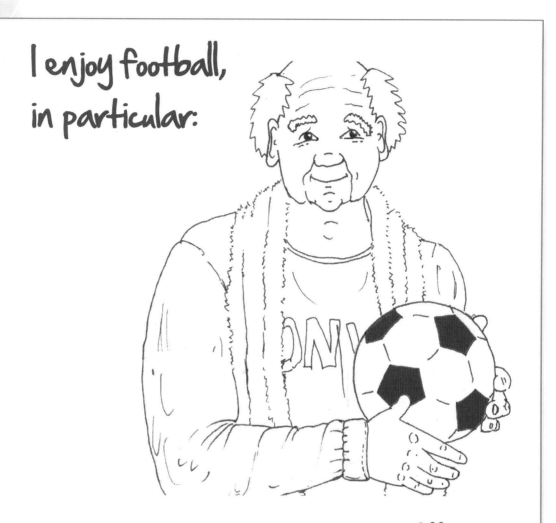

I enjoy football, in particular:

Aston Villa

You could include team strip, flags or colours.

# I enjoy reading newspapers and non-fiction books

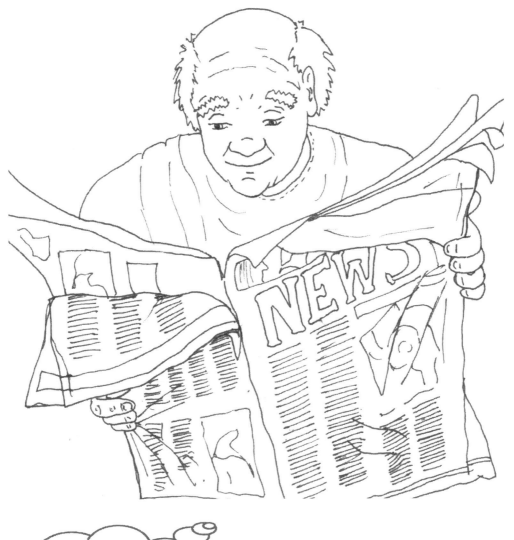

Put in the titles of some favourite books, newspapers, characters or quotes.

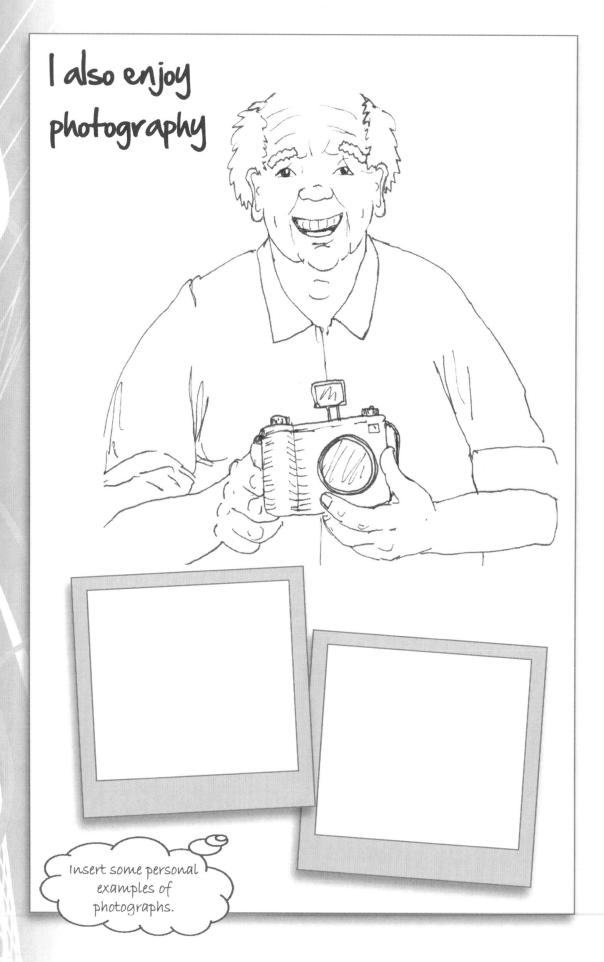

# I also enjoy photography

Insert some personal examples of photographs.

I am a sociable man and I enjoy chatting with family and friends

I am always the life and soul of a party, enjoy telling jokes and doing impersonations

Add a favourite joke or character.

Routledge
Taylor & Francis Group

# I would like to go to Australia and try sky diving

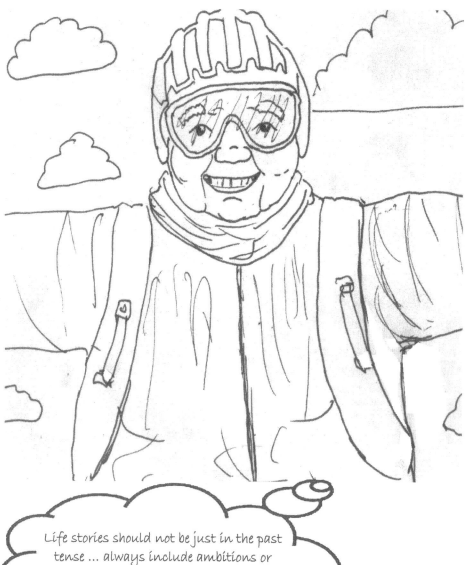

# Information signs

**Recording information about yourself and your life now**

## Skills

- Choosing likes/dislikes
- Typing text
- Deleting
- Saving work
- Opening files
- Printing
- Choosing photos/pictures
- Making text boxes

- Click and drag
- Searching online
- Cutting and pasting
- Scanning photos
- Inserting pictures

> Using symbols and pictures can aid understanding. Check with participants which is easier for them and which they prefer.

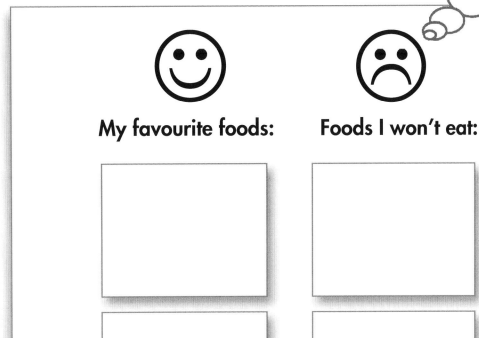

**My favourite foods:**

**Foods I won't eat:**

> Information signs need to be clear to all users. Useful symbols can be found in Word using Webdings. Choose Insert/Symbol/Font/Webdings.

Routledge
Taylor & Francis Group

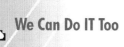

# Making signs

## Skills

- Recognising symbols

- Selecting symbols

- Resizing

- Changing background colour

- Printing

- Laminating

# Making signs

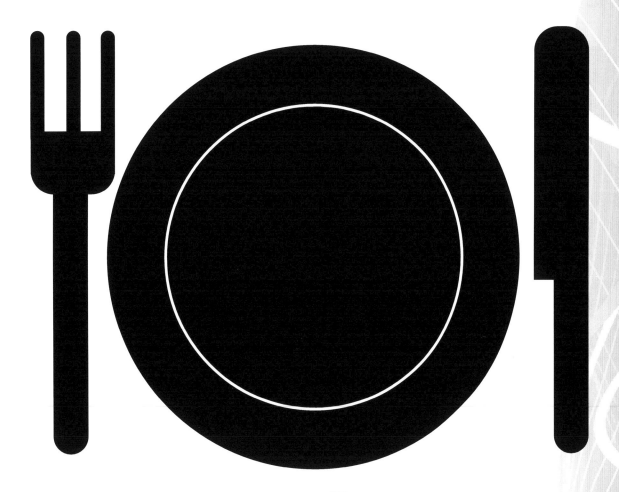

Think about the colour of the
sign against the background.
Black on yellow is considered the
best visual contrast.

Routledge
Taylor & Francis Group

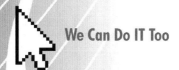

# Photographic menus

## Skills

- Digital photography
- Naming foods
- Typing text
- Selecting font
- Inserting text
- Inserting photographs

- Scanning
- Saving work
- Opening files
- Printing
- Laminating

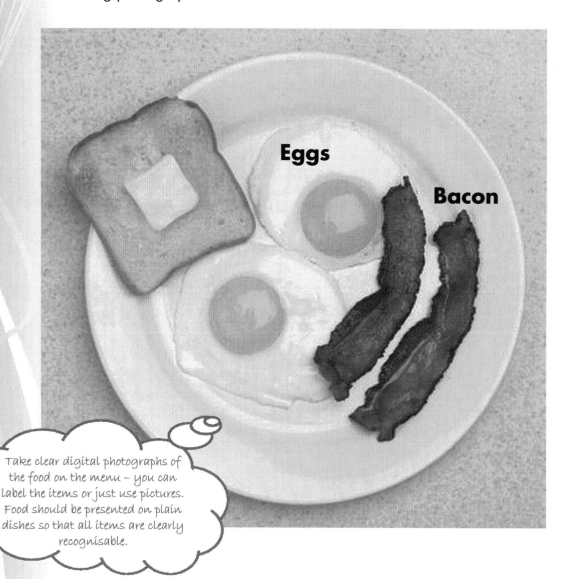

Take clear digital photographs of the food on the menu – you can label the items or just use pictures. Food should be presented on plain dishes so that all items are clearly recognisable.

114

# Calendar

| | Monday | Tuesday | Wednesday | Thursday | Friday | Saturday | Sunday |
|---|---|---|---|---|---|---|---|
| 10am | 🚌 | | | | | Lie in | Church |
| 11am | Shopping | | | | | | |
| 12.30pm | 🍽️ | 🍽️ | 🍽️ | 🍽️ | 🍽️ | 🍽️ Pub | 🍽️ Bob's |
| 2pm | | | Art group | | | | |
| 4pm | 🚗 Picked up by Cathy | | | | | | |

Laminate plain calendars that can be written on each week or use 'hook and loop' fastening tape to add pictures.

Use words or symbols depending on the individual. Differentiate the weekend or regular daily events by adding coloured shading.

Routledge
Taylor & Francis Group

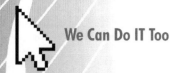

# Daily timetable

## Skills

- Talking about activities

- Identifying times of day

- Orientation to day/date/month

- Sequencing events

- Typing text

- Resizing font

- Selecting symbols or pictures

- Inserting pictures

- Digital photography

- Inserting tables

| Time | Monday |
|------|--------|
| 8.30am | Claire comes to help with shower and breakfast |
| | Write the time or mark on a clock face. |
| | You can use a mixture of text, symbols and pictures or make a plain template, laminate and stick pictures on using 'hook and loop' fastenings. |
| 2pm | |
| 3pm | Pick grandchildren up from school with Jim |

# Family tree

## Skills

Reminiscence, dialogue about family, choosing and naming photographs, making a timeline, typing text, changing fonts, inserting text boxes, scanning photos, inserting photos

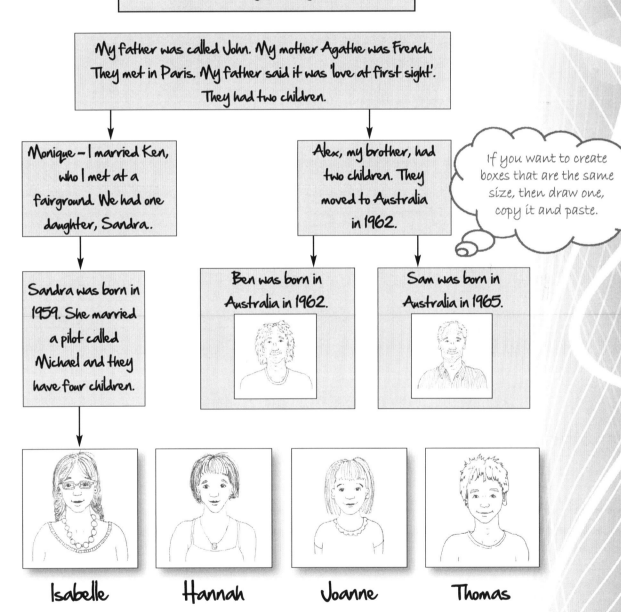

My name is Monique Sadler. Here is my family tree.

My father was called John. My mother Agathe was French. They met in Paris. My father said it was 'love at first sight'. They had two children.

Monique – I married Ken, who I met at a fairground. We had one daughter, Sandra.

Alex, my brother, had two children. They moved to Australia in 1962.

If you want to create boxes that are the same size, then draw one, copy it and paste.

Sandra was born in 1959. She married a pilot called Michael and they have four children.

Ben was born in Australia in 1962.

Sam was born in Australia in 1965.

Isabelle

Hannah

Joanne

Thomas

Routledge
Taylor & Francis Group

# Newsletter

## Skills

- Talking about content
- Interviewing
- Choosing styles
- Making columns
- Inserting text
- Inserting Word art
- Taking photos
- Inserting photos or pictures
- Printing
- Distributing

**You could use the Word art feature to make a title bar for your newsletter.**

Pick a font size and style that suits the nature of the newsletter.

Try not to use more than two styles of font in one newsletter – perhaps one style for headings and another for main text.

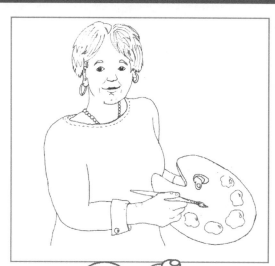

Include a variety of text and pictures, news, reports, future events.

Work in columns (you can insert columns from the Format menu).

# Glossary

This glossary gives brief explanations of some of the terms used in the book. We have not always used dictionary definitions and we have included explanations that will help you to use this book.

You may want to use some of these definitions to explain to clients how the computer works. You will notice that there are sometimes different words for the same thing, for example monitor and screen. When working with people with dementia it is a good idea to decide on one word and stick to it to avoid confusion.

There are internet dictionaries such as the one at www.netlingo.com (accessed February 2011) that explain computer and internet jargon.

**Accessibility** The way in which designers make things (including computers) easier to use for people with specific difficulties such as sensory impairment or problems with movement.

**Antivirus software** A program that detects and destroys viruses. This software may come as standard with your computer or you may need to buy it. Computer viruses are being developed all the time, so it is important to keep your antivirus software updated.

**Camera** Any device that takes photographs. Cameras can now be found on mobile phones and many can make short movies.

**Click** A function to make the mouse work. Pressing either button on the mouse makes a small 'click' sound.

**Clip art** Standard free images that are available to use via Microsoft applications.

**Copyright** A legal term meaning that someone owns the image or text. Most images on the internet are copyright and therefore cannot be used by anyone else.

**Desktop computer** A desktop computer is one that sits on a desktop. It usually comes in separate parts: a box or processing unit attached to a monitor or screen, with 'input devices' such as a keyboard and mouse.

**Desktop** The opening screen on your computer. A place where you keep important things (as on an office desktop). It contains icons that allow you to start your favourite programs.

**Digital camera/digital photography** Older cameras use film, which usually has to be developed and printed professionally. Digital cameras store the photographs on a memory card. The photographs can be easily copied from the camera to a computer.

**Dongle** A small piece of hardware that looks like a memory stick and enables your computer to use certain software (such as an internet connection).

**Download** To transfer a file (text, picture, video) from the internet (website or email) to your computer.

**Email** The usual name for electronic mail, messages that are sent from one computer to another via the internet. You need an email account with an email address to send and receive email.

**External hard drive** A device that plugs into your computer where you can store files and work you have done. It is useful because you can easily detach it from the computer.

**Font** The style of the text. There are many different typefaces, or fonts, available that can give a different appearance to the words displayed.

**Freezing** A term to describe what happens when the program you are using on the computer suddenly stops responding.

**Google** The most popular search engine on the web.

**Googlemail** An email service provided by Google.

**Hardware** Physical items of kit that make the computer work, for example the screen or monitor.

**Icon** A small, cartoon-like picture or symbol that represents something on the computer. Computer designers like to use icons as they save space that would be taken up by words.

**ICT** An abbreviation for information and communication technologies. It encompasses computers and telephones.

**Internet** The system by which computers are linked together. The internet allows people to use email and view websites.

**Internet connection** A way of linking your computer to the internet. This is done via telephone lines, but the connection can be 'wireless'.

**Internet service provider (ISP)** A commercial company that provides your connection to the internet via a telephone line.

**IT** An abbreviation for information technology, meaning anything to do with computers.

**Joystick** An input device that is often used with games. Joysticks can be useful for people who have difficulty using a mouse.

**Keyboard** It is like a typewriter and the keys are pressed to send letters and numbers to the computer.

**Laminator** A device for encapsulating paper in plastic.

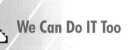 

**Laptop**  A computer that combines keyboard, screen and processor in one unit that can be easily carried around and used on your lap.

**Memory stick**  A small stick that plugs into your computer. You can copy your work – files and images – to the stick. It is useful if you need to take your work away from the computer.

**Mobile phone**  A phone that is designed to be taken out of the home. Mobile phones rely on signals and therefore often do not work in tunnels etc.

**Monitor**  The computer screen.

**Mouse**  An input device that controls the cursor or pointer on the screen.

**Online**  A shorthand word meaning 'on the internet'.

**Operating system**  The system that makes your computer work. Often this is Windows.

**PDF**  Stands for portable document format. A way of printing a document to an electronic format that retains the document styles and is difficult to edit.

**Pointer/cursor**  The symbol on the screen that is controlled by the mouse.

**Presentation**  A way of working on the computer that allows you to show one page after another. Pages in presentation software are often called slides.

**Printer toner**  'Ink' for the printer.

**Printer**  A device that allows you to make paper copies of what is on the screen. There are various types of printer.

**Program**  A piece of software that has been created to let you perform a specific activity on the computer. For example, there are programs for writing letters etc. (word processor), for doing calculations (spreadsheets) and for changing pictures.

**Projector**  A device that projects the screen on to a wall. It is useful when working in groups as it allows everyone to see what is happening on the computer.

**PS/2**  A way of plugging in devices.

**QWERTY keyboard**  A standard keyboard found in offices. QWERTY are the letters on the top row.

**Rollerball/trackball mouse** A type of mouse where the ball is on the top instead of underneath. Instead of moving the whole mouse around, users move the ball to make the cursor or pointer move across the screen.

**Scanner** A device that allows the computer to make a picture of the content on a piece of paper.

**Screen** Another word for monitor.

**Search engine/searching the internet** A search engine is a specialist website that acts as a giant index for all websites. Google is the best known. You type a word or phrase into a search box and click on the search button. A list of websites that are relevant to the word or phrase will be displayed.

**Security** Some people will try to access your computer illegally. They may want to find out personal or financial information about you, or break the computer. There are various pieces of software and hardware that are designed to protect your computer.

**Shift key** The key on the keyboard with an arrow on it. Keeping it pressed at the same time as pressing a letter key will produce a capital letter. Its name dates from the old days of typewriters.

**Skype** A commercial service that allows you to speak to another person via your computers.

**Slide show** A type of presentation that shows one screen after another.

**Software** The instructions that control what the computer does.

**Text** The writing on the computer screen.

**Touch screen** A special screen that allows users to control the cursor and display by touching the screen.

**Touchpad** An input device usually seen on laptops. Moving your finger around the pad controls the movement of the cursor or pointer.

**Upgrades** Software producers always want to make improvements. Whenever they change their software they issue an upgrade. This usually has to be downloaded from their website and often has to be paid for.

**USB** A type of plug to attach devices to your computer.

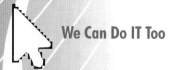 

**USB board**  A board with lots of USB sockets.

**Video**  Moving images captured digitally.

**Voice recordings**  Recordings made through the computer or a recording device.

**Webcam**  A small camera attached to a computer that shows live images from the internet.

**Website**  A small area of the world wide web that has a specific address. The address usually starts with www.

**WiFi**  Wireless access to the internet.

**Wireless router**  A box that plugs into a telephone socket and allows you to have wireless connection to the internet within your building.

**Word art**  A function in Microsoft Word programs that allows you to add fancy pre-set text styles, usually as headings in your work.

**Word processing**  A program that allows you to manipulate text.

**YouTube website**  A specialist website where people upload and share short videos.

# Programs and applications

## Internet browsers

Internet browsers allow you to view websites. The most common are Internet Explorer, Mozilla Firefox and Safari. In addition to displaying websites, browsers will also allow you to save favourites, look at your 'history' (a list of sites you have looked at) and change your 'home page' (the page you see first when you open up the browser).

## Presentation software

Presentation software such as Microsoft PowerPoint is designed for people giving presentations. However, these software packages are useful for producing other things such as life story books and automatic slide shows. They are very useful when you are using a lot of images. Each component – images or text – is in its own 'box' and can be moved around independently of the other components on the page. It is also possible to link the pages to each other through action buttons, animations and transitions.

## Word processing

Word-processing packages such as Microsoft Word allow you to manipulate text. You can format text in various ways – size, style, font, colour, spacing, columns, tables etc. You can also add pictures.

# Techniques and tips

This section highlights and explains some of the techniques we have found useful.

## Backing up your work

Computers sometimes break down. It is also relatively easy to accidentally delete or change files that you meant to keep. It would be sad to lose things that have been created by your group. Backing up data simply means copying the files and folders from your computer and keeping the copies somewhere else. This could be on a memory stick or an external hard drive. It would be a good idea to keep the back-up somewhere away from the main computer.

## Cursor/pointer

When explaining the different things you can do with the computer, it is worth looking at the different ways the cursor or pointer is displayed. For example:

- When giving a command, such as opening an application or using a menu, the cursor is an arrow.

- When working with text the cursor is an I-beam.

- When hovering over a link on a webpage it turns into a hand.

- When manipulating images the cursor changes to indicate moving, resizing or cropping.

## Cut and paste

Cut and paste is a major feature of word processing that can also be used in nearly all computer programs. The idea is to take a feature of your work (for example, a piece of text or an image), copy it or cut it out temporarily to the computer and then 'paste' it into a different document or another location within the same document. First, the item has to be 'selected' (highlighted or clicked on), then the command to cut or copy given, and finally you click where you want to paste and give the command to paste.

## Drag and drop

Drag and drop is an important technique for people using computers. If you click on an object such as an image and hold the mouse button down you will be able to move the image around the screen. When you release the button the image is 'dropped' where your cursor is. A good way to practise 'drag and drop' is to play the game Solitaire on the computer. Some special types of mouse and some accessibility settings allow you to drag and drop without holding down the mouse button.

# Dual control

When working with people who are not confident using computers, it is often helpful to do some of the work for them. To avoid having to lean over them or taking the mouse away, think about having an additional mouse attached to the computer. The person with dementia is still in control, but it is possible for you to say, for example, 'Shall I choose the colour for you? I'll move the pointer to this colour – now you click and the colour will change.' The person with dementia is still in charge and understands that what you and they are doing makes a change to the screen. But the stress of carrying out every different mouse move and click is removed.

# Keyboard shortcuts, toolbars or menus

Most computers and programs will offer a variety of ways to do the same thing. For example, saving a document can be done either through an icon on a toolbar, through the menus or via a keyboard shortcut (holding down the Ctrl button at the same time as the S key). The people you are working with may be used to using different methods. All are valid. If you are working with people who are new to computers it is probably a good idea to be consistent and to use only the menus or toolbars, where possible.

# Manipulating images

Images can be inserted from a variety of sources: directly from a camera, from scanned images saved on your computer, from free clip art, from images saved from the web (but be careful about copyright). In most packages you can insert images, although they will usually be the wrong size. Most packages will let you resize, move and crop images. Usually this is done by selecting the image (when the image is selected a box will appear around it) and manipulating it by means of the 'handles' on the box.

# Organising files and folders

It is a good idea to organise your files on the computer in a systematic way to ensure that you can find items again. If you are working with a group, it might be a good idea to keep all the files to do with one project together. If you are working with individuals it might be worth keeping all the files created or used by each individual together. You can create a new folder and name it for each individual or project. When you save a file or download an image remember to save into the correct folder.

# Print and print preview

Most applications will enable you to 'preview' what your document will look like when you print it out. This is particularly useful in helping to save on coloured toner! You could also investigate different printing options such as printing on both sides of the paper if your printer allows it or changing the page layout to print out in landscape format.

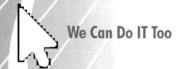

## Right click

If you are ever stuck and do not know how to do something, it is always worth clicking on the right mouse button. This will give you a short menu of functions that you can do at that particular part of the screen. Try it and see!

## Save and Save As

The most important thing you can do is to save your work regularly. Saving a file means giving it a name and location (a file name and a location within a particular folder on your computer). Once a piece of work is saved it can be opened again and you can continue to work. If you do not save and power is lost, or the computer freezes or crashes, you will lose your work.

Save As allows you to save a copy of your work with a different name. This feature is very useful if you want to make two different pieces of work that are the same apart from (for example) a name or date. Create the first document with 'John' at the top called letterJ.doc and then Save As letterM.doc and change John to Mary.

## Selecting text and objects

Before you can do anything to a piece of text or an image you need to 'select' it. This means telling the computer that you are only interested in that particular bit of text or image.

If you are working with a text box or an image, simply clicking on the box will select it. You know that the object is selected because a thick box appears around it.

To select individual words or sections of text you click on the beginning of the text and hold the button down as you move the mouse to the end of it. This action 'highlights' the text.

Once an object is selected, you can tell the computer to change it: move it, change fonts, colours, size etc.

## Text boxes

Text boxes are used in many word-processing and presentation software applications. If you create a text box you can move the whole box separately from other text on the page. You can also add borders or background colours. Text boxes are used in a similar way to images and can be resized and moved around easily.

# References

**Alzheimer's Society** 'About dementia. Statistics'
www.alzheimers.org.uk

**Banerjee S** (2009) *The Use of Antipsychotic Medication for People with Dementia: Time for Action. A Report for the Minister of State for Care Services*, Department of Health, London
www.dh.gov.uk

**Care Quality Commission** (formerly Healthcare Commission)
www.cqc.ord.uk

**Department of Constitutional Affairs**, tel. 0207 210 0025
www.dca.gov.uk/legal-policy/mental-capacity

**Department of Health** (2001) *National Service Framework for Older People*, No. 23633
www.dh.gov.uk

**Health and Safety Executive** (2006) 'Five steps to risk assessment'
www.hse.gov.uk/pubns/indg163.pdf

**Healthcare Commission** (2009) *Equality in Later Life: A National Study of Older People's Mental Health Services*
www.cqc.org.uk/_db/_documents/Equality_in_later_life.pdf

**Housing21 Dementia Voice**
www.housing21.co.uk/corporate-information/housing-21-dementia-voice/

**Mckeown J, Clarke A & Repper J** (2006) 'Life story work in health and social care: systematic literature review', *Journal of Advanced Nursing*, 55 (2), pp237–47.

**Mental Capacity Act** (2005)
www.legislation.gov.uk/ukpga/2005/9/part/1

**NHS** (2008) 'Advance decision to refuse treatment proforma', National End of Life Care Programme
www.endoflifecareforadults.nhs.uk/assets/downloads/ADRT_form.pdf

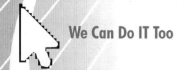 

**NESTA (National Endowment for Science, Technology and the Arts)**
www.nesta.org.uk/about_us

**Office of the Public Guardian**
www.publicguardian.gov.uk

**Parr S, Pound C, Byng S & Long B** (2004) *The Stroke and Aphasia Handbook*, Connect Ltd, London.

**Smith M, Kolanowski A, Buettner L & Buckwalter K** (2009) 'Beyond bingo: meaningful activities for persons with dementia in nursing homes', *Annals of Long-Term Care*, 17 (7), pp22–30.

All websites accessed February 2011.

## Useful addresses and organisations

**AbilityNet**
www.abilitynet.org.uk

**Alzheimer's Society**, Devon House, 58 St Katharine's Way, London E1W 1LB
www.alzheimers.org.uk

**Charity Commission**
www.charity.commission.gov.uk

**NetLingo**
www.netlingo.com

**Stroke Association**, Stroke House, 240 City Road, London EC1V 2PR
www.stroke.org.uk